Migraines Demystified

Your Snarky, Science-Backed Survival Guide

Ken Konet, M.Ed., MBA

As an individual with firsthand experience managing migraines, I am committed to assisting you in finding an effective solution for yourself or for your patient.

Copyright

Migraines Demystified: Your Snarky, Science-Backed Survival Guide

Published by Humbolton, LLC; Dallas, Texas

Cover Design: Isabella Green

Interior Design: Isabella Green

Illustrations/Infographics: Created with the help of AI.

Clinical Contributions & Medical Review: Elliott James, APRN, MSN, CMRD

ISBN (Paperback): 978-1-966703-20-4

ISBN (eBook): Amazon

First Edition, 2026
Printed in the United States of America

Table of Contents

Introduction: Welcome to the Club Nobody Wants to Join

Let's get one thing straight right from the start. If you picked up this book, chances are you or someone you love is a member of the world's most exclusive, least fun, and most painfully misunderstood club: The Migraine Warriors. Our secret handshake is a pained squint in a moderately lit room, our motto is "No, it's not just a headache," and our initiation rite involves questioning all your life choices while clutching an ice pack to your skull like it's a religious artifact.

So, welcome. I'm sorry you're here, but I'm damn glad we found each other.

If you're like me, you've been on the receiving end of a tidal wave of well-meaning but utterly useless advice. It's a veritable bingo card of nonsense.

"Have you tried drinking more water?" Check.

"You should just relax more. Have you tried yoga?" Check. And yes, I've tried yoga. It's hard to find your zen when you're worried the downward dog will make your brain explode.

"Maybe you're just stressed." Check. Well, I wasn't, but I am now. Thanks.

And the fan-favorite, the one that makes you want to flip a table: "Oh, I get bad headaches too."

Let's be clear: comparing a migraine to a headache is like comparing a house cat to a velociraptor. They might share a few superficial similarities, but one is a cute nuisance and the other is a prehistoric predator actively trying to dismantle you from the inside out. A headache is a bad day. A migraine is a full-system neurological revolt, a chaotic, unsanctioned rave your brain decides to throw, complete with a throbbing bassline, strobe lights you can't turn off, and a bouncer who's decided your own consciousness is no longer on the VIP list.

This book is the antidote to that nonsense. This is your official, science-backed, snark-filled permission slip to tell the next person who offers you a sip of water to politely, or not-so-politely, take a long walk off a short pier.

This isn't a dry medical textbook that could bore a rock into a coma. And it's not a wellness blog promising a cure-all via kale smoothie. This is a survival manual written by someone who has studied the enemy and fought it in the trenches. I get it. I've lived it. I've had my day, my week, my month derailed by a brain that decided to go rogue.

📖 A Note From the Author: Why I'm Not Just the Guy Who Wrote This Book

I need to tell you something before we get into the science, the strategies, and the snark. Something I want you to hold onto especially on the days when you feel like you've tried everything, seen everyone, and gotten nowhere. I spent nearly five years fighting this battle without a real answer. Five years of waking up and wondering if today was going to be a "functional human" day or a "dark room, ice pack, do not speak to me" day. I saw eight different doctors. Eight.

I even went to the Mayo Clinic -- yes, that Mayo Clinic, the one people fly across the country to see when no one else has figured it out. I tried medications, injections, lifestyle overhauls, specialists of every stripe. Some things helped a little. Nothing helped enough. Nothing lasted. And here's the part that still gets me: I was being treated for migraines. For years. By smart, well-meaning, genuinely competent doctors. Turns out, my neck had been quietly plotting against me the whole time.

The real culprit -- multilevel cervical degeneration, bone spurs pressing on nerves, a structural problem that was generating migraine-level head pain from the neck up -- was sitting right there in my old MRI and CT scans. Hiding in plain sight. It took me uploading those scans into an AI tool and asking a simple question -- "What could be causing all of my headache, migraine, hyperacusis, vomiting, etc.?" -- to finally get a roadmap that made sense. The AI flagged cervical involvement immediately and suggested potential solutions. I brought those insights to a surgeon. We did diagnostic testing. And for the first time in almost five years, I got a preview of my old life back.

I haven't had my surgery yet as I write this. But the diagnostic shots alone -- the ones we used to confirm the source -- gave me a window of relief I hadn't felt in years. I remembered what it was like to just be a person, without the constant background noise of pain. And that was enough to make me genuinely, unreservedly excited about my future for the first time in a very long time.

So why am I telling you this in the introduction, instead of just getting to the good stuff? Because I want you to know two things. **First:** if you've been fighting this for years and still don't have answers, you are not crazy, you are not weak, and you are not a medical mystery. You may just have the wrong map. **Second:** the solution -- wherever it comes from, whether it's a new medication, a structural diagnosis, a lifestyle change, or a conversation with an AI at midnight, and a knowledgeable physician -- exists. I promise you it exists. You just haven't found it yet.

That's what this book is for. Let's go find it.

We're going to tear down the mysteries surrounding this debilitating condition. We'll cover everything from the "classic" skull-splitters that feel like an ice pick is being introduced to your eyeball, to the weird, wild, and criminally misdiagnosed cousins of migraine. We're talking about the conditions that other books gloss over -- the neuralgias, like Occipital and Trigeminal, that send lightning bolts of pain zinging from your neck and face. We're going to explore why your neck sometimes feels like it's actively plotting against you and how ordinary, everyday light and sound can transform into instruments of physical assault.

This book reframes migraine management from a frustrating guessing game into a strategic mission. It's engineered for how a brain in pain actually works -- with stunning, full-page infographics that explain complex science in a single glance, one-page cheat sheets you can snap a photo of for later, and bite-sized, actionable intel that you can absorb even when your brain feels like scrambled eggs.

Because let's be honest, when you're in the throes of an attack, the last thing you have the energy for is a 1,000-word essay on the pathophysiology of calcitonin gene-related peptide (CGRP). You need answers, you need them now, and you need them to be clear.

So, what exactly did you just get yourself into?

Inside this guide, you will find:

- The Migraine Multiverse, Unlocked: A full-color, visually-driven tour of every type of attack, from the common offenders to the criminally overlooked neuralgia-induced episodes that leave doctors scratching their heads.
- The "Four Horsemen" Blueprint: Forget abstract science. We'll introduce you to the four key players in your personal migraine apocalypse with a battle plan to help you predict, intercept, and outmaneuver attacks in real-time.
- Evidence-Backed Arsenals: No more endless lists of medications. We'll map out your treatment paths -- from classic meds and CGRP rockstars to next-gen neuromodulation devices -- on a clear, infographic "Ladder of Therapies" so you know what to ask your doctor for and when.
- Your Personal "Brain Dashboard": We'll give you the tools -- including a complete Trigger Matrix and a DIY diary template -- to spot your unique attack patterns in under 60 seconds a day. You'll become the Sherlock Holmes of your own brain.
- Life-Proof Playbooks: This is where the rubber meets the road. You'll get no-nonsense scripts for navigating tricky conversations with your boss, your partner, and your doctor. We've even included a "Caregiver Quick-Start Guide" for the people who love you but have no idea what to do when you're down for the count.
- **Clinical Insider Notes:** This book isn't just one patient's perspective. Woven throughout these pages, you'll find clinical sidebars and medical review contributed by Elliott James, APRN, MSN, CMRD — a board-certified neurology Nurse Practitioner who also happens to be one of the author's own healthcare providers. His contributions bridge the gap between what you experience as a patient and what your provider is thinking on the other side of the exam table. It's the kind of clinical insight most books can't give you, because most books don't have an actual provider in the room while they're being written.

By blending cutting-edge neuroscience with irreverent humor and concrete, actionable steps, Migraines Demystified is designed to arm you -- and your entire support crew -- with the clarity, tools, and confidence to finally, hopefully help you to reclaim your life.

♥□ A Word to Everyone Else in the Room

If you picked up this book because someone you love handed it to you, or because you're trying to understand what your patient, your employee, your friend, or your family member is going through -- welcome. Pull up a chair. This book is for you too.

You didn't ask to be part of this story. You didn't sign up for cancelled plans, darkened rooms, whispered conversations, and the particular helplessness of watching someone you care about suffer while there's nothing you can visibly do to fix it. That is genuinely hard. And it doesn't get acknowledged enough.

So let me say it plainly: your presence matters more than you know. The partner who creates the migraine cave without being asked. The friend who texts "no pressure, feel better" instead of guilt-tripping over a cancelled dinner. The doctor who takes the time to connect the dots between a patient's neck pain and their "migraines." The coworker who turns down the office lights without making it a big deal. These things are not small. To someone in pain, they are everything.

Throughout this book, you'll find content written directly for you -- not just instructions for the sufferer on how to manage their relationships, but real guidance, in plain language, for the people in the orbit of this condition. Look for the ♥□ Inner Circle and □ Clinical Note callouts -- those are yours.

You don't have to understand every chapter. You don't have to become a neurologist. You just have to want to help. And since you're already holding this book, you've already passed that test.

One more thing before we move on. Throughout this book, you'll find clinical sidebars and medical review notes contributed by **Elliott James, APRN, MSN, CMRD** — a board-certified Advanced Practice Registered Nurse specializing in neurology and movement disorders. Elliott isn't just some random expert I cold-called for a blurb. He's one of my own healthcare providers — part of the team that has been managing my care through this entire journey. When I decided this book needed a clinical voice to complement the patient perspective, the choice was obvious. His contributions bring the kind of real-world clinical insight that you can only get from someone who actually sits across from patients every day and helps them navigate this condition. You'll see his work marked with the □ symbol throughout.

How to Use This Book: Your Survival Strategy

This book was not designed to be read cover-to-cover like a novel (unless you're a masochist who enjoys reading about pain, in which case, you do you). It was designed by thinking like an instructional designer -- someone whose entire job is to make information as clear, accessible, and usable as humanly possible. Think of it as a reference manual, a field guide, or a military-grade toolkit. Your mission is to use it strategically.

Here's the breakdown of your new arsenal:

The book is organized into five distinct parts, moving you logically from knowledge to action:

- **Part I: UNDERSTAND (The First Principles)** This is your foundational knowledge. Your mission here, should you choose to accept it, is to finally understand what the hell is happening inside your skull. We'll cover Migraines 101, explore the different types of attacks (the "Migraine Multiverse"), and dissect the anatomy of an attack from the first weird yawn to the brain-fog hangover. Start here if you're new to this world or if you want to arm yourself with the science to shut down the next person who tells you to "just take an aspirin."
- **Part II: ANTICIPATE (Decode the Signals)** This section is about becoming a migraine psychic. No crystal ball required -- just data. We'll dive deep into the trigger minefield, teaching you not just what your triggers are, but how they stack up like dominoes to cause an attack. Then, we'll help you build your personal "Migraine Dashboard" using diaries, apps, and wearables to get those crucial early warnings. If you feel like your migraines come out of nowhere, this part is for you.
- **Part III: ACT (The Two-Tier Toolkit)** This is the emergency response section. This is where you come when an attack is

imminent or already in full swing. It's split into two no-nonsense chapters: The Acute Attack Playbook (how to shut it down FAST) and The Preventive Arsenal (how to build your long-term defenses). No fluff, just action. If you're in pain right now, skip everything else and come straight here.

- **Part IV: THRIVE (Life Beyond the Pain)** You are more than your migraine. This section is dedicated to proving it. We'll cover everything from "lifestyle engineering" (migraine-proofing your home and office) and managing the mental health doom loop (anxiety, guilt, isolation) to navigating the real world of work, school, and relationships with scripts and strategies. Come here when you're ready to move from just surviving to actually living again.
- **Part V: ADVOCATE (Bigger Than One Brain)** This is where you become the expert in the room -- especially when that room has a doctor in it. We'll teach you how to navigate the infuriating labyrinth of doctors and insurance, how to spot comorbidities and copycats that might be complicating your case, and we'll give you a hopeful glimpse into the future of migraine research. This section is for when you're ready to take charge of your healthcare journey.

The Field Manual (Your Tear-Out Toolkit)

At the end of the book, you'll find the Field Manual—a collection of one-page tools designed to be torn out, printed, or saved to your phone:

The Migraine Phase Wheel: A color-coded poster to hang on your fridge.

The Trigger Matrix: A blank template to track your personal landmines.

The Medication Family Tree: An infographic to make sense of your pharmacy haul.

The Care-Partner One-Pager: A 5-step guide to hand to anyone who's ever asked, "What can I do to help?"

The Doctor Visit Planner: A fillable form to ensure your next appointment is ruthlessly efficient.

Read this book any way you want. Start at the beginning, jump to the middle, or go straight to the Field Manual. My only job is to provide the map.

A final word before we dive in. Living with migraines can feel incredibly isolating. It's a silent, invisible battle that few people understand. But you are not alone. There is an entire army of us out here, fighting the same fight, armed with ice packs and an unshakeable, if sometimes weary, sense of resilience. This book is a tribute to that strength. It's a tool, a guide, and a reminder that even on the darkest days, there is hope, there is help, and there is a community that has your back. **Now, let's get to work.**

⚠□ WHEN TO SEEK EMERGENCY CARE

This book is about understanding and managing migraines. It is not a substitute for emergency medicine. Call 911 or go to your nearest emergency room immediately if you experience any of the following:

• The worst headache of your life, sudden and severe ("thunderclap") • Headache with fever, stiff neck, confusion, seizures, or rash • Weakness, numbness, or paralysis on one side of your body • Sudden vision loss, slurred speech, or difficulty understanding language • Headache following a head injury, especially with worsening symptoms

These symptoms can indicate stroke, meningitis, aneurysm, or other life-threatening conditions that mimic or co-occur with migraine. When in doubt, do not wait. Err on the side of the emergency room.

Chapter 1: Migraines 101

Your Brain's Electrical Rebellion

Let's kick this off by getting one thing tattooed on our collective consciousness. Say it with me now, out loud if you have to, maybe even get it printed on a mug: Migraines. Are. Not. Just. Headaches.

There. I feel better already.

If you've ever described your symptoms to someone—the one-sided agony, the nausea, the feeling that sunlight has become your mortal enemy—only to be met with, "Oh, I get bad headaches too," then you know the unique brand of rage I'm talking about.

A migraine is a neurological betrayal.

It's a full-system, DEFCON 1, electrical rebellion staged by the three-pound tyrant living in your skull. It's every nerve ending in your head deciding to file a grievance at the same time, while the pain department cranks the volume to eleven and the nausea department sends a sympathy gift nobody asked for.

So, this chapter is our ground zero. Our boot camp. Before we can learn to fight the enemy, we need to understand it. We need to look it in its multifaceted, pain-inducing eye and see it for what it truly is: a bona-fide, card-carrying, complex neuro-immune disorder. To do that, we need to meet the ringleaders of this whole sordid affair.

The Four Horsemen of the typical migraine apocalypse.

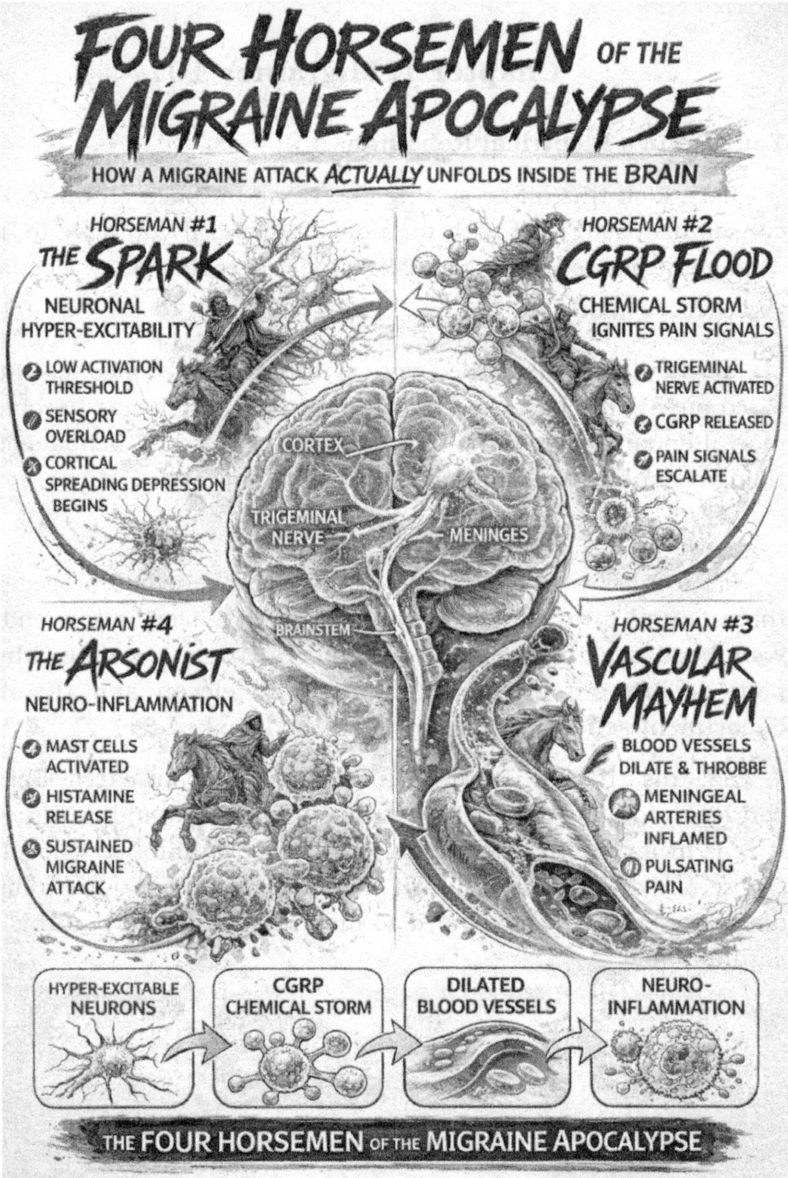

Image made with the help of AI

Meet Horseman #1: The Spark (Neuronal Hyper-excitability)

The first horseman isn't the pain itself. It's the spark that lights the fuse. The scientific term is neuronal hyper-excitability, which is a fancy way of saying your brain is a high-strung, over-caffeinated overachiever.

Imagine your brain's nerve cells (neurons) are like a car alarm system. In a non-migraine brain, the alarm only goes off when someone actually breaks a window. It's appropriate. It's proportional. In a migraine brain, that alarm is set to "ridiculously sensitive." A leaf falls on the hood? ALARM. A strong gust of wind? ALARM. Someone looks at it funny? FULL-BLOWN, WAKE-THE-NEIGHBORS ALARM.

Your neurons have a lower-than-average activation threshold. They fire off electrical signals at the slightest provocation. This is why common, everyday stimuli that other people barely notice---a flickering fluorescent light, the perfume counter at a department store, a slight change in air pressure---can feel like a full-frontal assault to you. Your brain isn't just noticing these things; it's treating them as an existential threat.

This state of hyper-excitability is what sets the stage for the infamous Cortical Spreading Depression (CSD). Despite its depressing name, CSD isn't an emotional state; it's a physical phenomenon. It's a slow-moving, self-propagating wave of intense electrical activity that creeps across the surface of your brain (the cortex) like a ripple in a pond, typically at a snail's pace of 3-5 millimeters per minute.

As this wave passes, it first causes neurons to fire like crazy, then leaves them exhausted and temporarily unable to function in its wake. If this wave travels across your visual cortex, you get a visual aura (the light show). If it crosses the sensory cortex, you might get tingling or numbness. CSD is the neurological event that starts the whole ugly cascade. It's the first domino to fall, and it's about to knock over a whole lot of its friends.

So, the first horseman isn't about pain. It's about potential. It's a brain that's fundamentally wired for rebellion, just waiting for the right excuse to start a riot.

For some people, these horsemen get called into action not just by a misfiring brain, but by something structural going on in the neck. We'll explore this important overlap in detail in Chapter 2.

Meet Horseman #2: The Chemical Warrior (The CGRP Flood)

Once the Spark has done its job and the CSD wave is on the move, the brain's alarm bells start ringing. This signals the trigeminal nerve---a massive cranial nerve with branches covering your face, sinuses, and the sensitive outer lining of the brain (the meninges)---to freak out. And when the trigeminal nerve freaks out, it unleashes its weapon of choice.

Enter the second horseman: a flood of a neuropeptide called Calcitonin Gene-Related Peptide, or CGRP.

If migraine were a disaster movie, CGRP is the monster. It's the big bad, the main villain, the chemical agent of chaos. For decades, scientists were chasing different theories, but the discovery of CGRP's central role was a seismic shift in our understanding. It's so important that the newest, most effective generation of migraine medications is designed specifically to block this one protein.

When the trigeminal nerve is activated by the CSD wave, it dumps CGRP all over the place. CGRP is a potent vasodilator, meaning it causes blood vessels to relax and expand. But its main job here is to act as a master of chemical warfare. It binds to receptors on the blood vessels of the meninges and on the nerve fibers themselves, kicking off two disastrous processes:

- It Causes Inflammation: CGRP makes blood vessels leaky and inflamed, spilling out other inflammatory substances into the surrounding tissue. This is a key source of the pain.
- It Transmits Pain Signals: CGRP is a world-class messenger of misery. It enhances the transmission of pain signals along the trigeminal nerve pathway, turning up the volume on the pain until it's all you can hear.

Think of it this way: the Spark (CSD) knocked on the door. The Chemical Warrior (CGRP) just blew the door off its hinges with a rocket launcher and is now setting up a command post in your cerebrum. This is why the pain feels so deep, so pervasive, and so inflammatory. It's not just in your head; it's a chemical siege.

Meet Horseman #3: The Conductor of Chaos (Vascular Mayhem)

For a long time, the prevailing theory was that migraines were purely a vascular problem---that blood vessels first constricted (causing aura) and then dilated (causing pain). This theory has since been demoted. We now know that the vascular changes aren't the cause of the migraine; they're a consequence of the neurological and chemical events orchestrated by the first two horsemen.

The third horseman, Vascular Mayhem, is the result of CGRP's handiwork.

Once CGRP has flooded the scene, the blood vessels around your brain, particularly the meningeal arteries, go into full-blown rave mode. They dilate, swell, and become painfully inflamed. The pulsing, throbbing, feels-like-my-heartbeat-is-in-my-eye pain that is so characteristic of migraine? You can thank this guy for that.

Every time your heart beats, it pushes blood through these now-swollen, hypersensitive vessels. Each pulse sends a wave of pain radiating through your skull. It's why lying perfectly still in a dark room is not just a preference; it's a survival strategy. Any movement, any light, any sound that activates your already-screaming nervous system makes the pulsing unbearable.

Meet Horseman #4: The Arsonist (Neuro-inflammation)

Meet the final horseman, the one who ensures the party doesn't stop. He's The Arsonist, and his game is neuro-inflammation. This isn't just about nerves firing and chemicals flooding. A full-blown migraine attack is an inflammatory event. Your brain's own immune cells, particularly cells called mast cells, get activated by the chaos. Mast cells are like tiny, localized SWAT teams that are supposed to respond to injury or allergens. But in a migraine, they get faulty intel. They see the CGRP flood and the vascular mayhem and think, "This is a five-alarm fire!"

So, they ride in and, in a misguided attempt to help, they make everything worse. They degranulate, which means they burst open and release their own potent cocktail of inflammatory chemicals, including histamine and serotonin. This is like throwing gasoline on a fire.

These new chemicals further irritate the nerve endings, make the blood vessels even leakier, and call in more immune cells to the party. This process, known as neurogenic inflammation, creates a self-sustaining cycle of pain and sensitization. It's why migraines can last for hours, or even days. The initial trigger may be long gone, but The Arsonist is still running around with a flamethrower, making sure the inflammatory fire keeps burning.

This is also why, after an attack, you feel like you've been hit by a truck. Your brain has just hosted a full-scale inflammatory war. The battlefield is littered with chemical residue, and the cleanup crew (your body's recovery systems) has a massive job ahead. That's the postdrome, or migraine hangover, which we'll get to later. So, there you have it. The Four Horsemen. A twitchy nervous system, a flood of chemical warriors, a throbbing vascular rave, and a brain on fire. It's a complex, brutal, and coordinated assault. It is not. just. a. headache.

The Difference Between a Bad Day and a Neurological Betrayal

Now that you've met the Four Horsemen, let's put this into context. Let's formally compare the common tension headache to the neurological thunderdome that is a migraine. Hand this chart to the next person who says they "get bad headaches too." See the difference? One is a minor inconvenience. The other is a multi-phase neurological event orchestrated by four very angry, very destructive Horsemen.

ACTION BOX: 60-Second Reality Check

Keep this in your back pocket for quick, science-backed clapbacks to the most infuriating migraine myths.

Myth #1: "It's just stress. You just need to relax." Reality Check: Stress is a trigger, not the cause. My brain is neurologically predisposed to overreact; a non-migraine brain under the same stress doesn't launch a full-scale chemical assault on itself.

Myth #2: "Have you tried drinking more water?" Reality Check: While dehydration can be a trigger for some, a migraine is a complex neuro-inflammatory event, not a simple case of thirst. No amount of water can stop a CGRP flood.

Myth #3: "It's all in your head." Reality Check: You're right, it is in my head---my brain, to be exact. It's a measurable, biological process involving electrical waves, inflammatory proteins, and vascular changes. It's as "in my head" as a stroke or epilepsy.

Myth #4: "Just take some painkillers and get on with it." Reality Check: Standard painkillers don't work on the complex mechanisms of a migraine. We need specific medications (like triptans or CGRP blockers) to target the neurological cascade, not just mask the pain.

Caregiver Intel Brief: What You Just Learned, In Plain English

For the partner, parent, friend, coworker, or anyone who just sat through the science above and is now wondering what any of it means for how to really help someone they love.

Here's the short version: a migraine is not a bad headache. It is a multi-stage neurological event involving electrical waves sweeping across the brain, a chemical flood that inflames blood vessels, and an immune response that can sustain pain for hours or even days. By the time a migraine sufferer tells you they can't function, their brain has already been under active assault for hours -- often before the pain even begins.

What this means for you, practically:

The person you love isn't being dramatic. They're not avoiding your plans, their responsibilities, or you. Their brain is in a genuine, measurable, biological crisis that they did not choose and cannot simply push through. "Just taking some painkillers" doesn't address the Four Horsemen any more than a band-aid addresses a broken arm.

The most helpful thing you can do during an attack is not to fix it -- you can't. It's to reduce the sensory load on an already overwhelmed nervous system. Darkness. Quiet. No questions. No new information. No suggestions. Just presence, calm, and the understanding that this will pass.

You are not helpless. You are exactly what they need: someone who gets it, shows up, and doesn't make it worse.

Throughout this book you'll find more specific guidance tailored to your role -- whether you're a partner, a parent, a friend, a coworker, or a clinician. Look for the ❤□ and □ callout boxes. They're written for you.

Chapter One Conclusion: Your Brain Isn't Broken---It's Just a Specialist

We've just waded through some heavy science, and it can be a lot to take in, especially when it's describing a battle happening inside your own body. So let's pause and reframe.

Knowing about the Four Horsemen isn't meant to scare you. It's meant to arm you. For too long, migraine sufferers have been told their pain isn't real, that it's psychological, or that they're just not tough enough. That's garbage. Your pain is real because the biological process causing it is real.

Understanding these mechanisms is the foundation of everything that follows. When you know the Spark makes your brain extra sensitive, you can engineer your environment. When you know CGRP is the key villain, you can understand why the new CGRP-blocking medications are revolutionary and advocate for them with your doctor. When you understand the roles of vascular changes and inflammation, you know this isn't just pain—it's a physical injury that requires rest and recovery.

This knowledge changes what you can do in a doctor's office, at a pharmacy counter, and in the middle of an attack. When you know the Spark makes your brain hyper-sensitive, you can engineer your environment to lower the voltage. When you know CGRP is the key chemical driver, you understand why the new CGRP-blocking medications exist and can ask your doctor about them with confidence. When you understand the roles of vascular changes and inflammation, you know this is not just pain—it is a physical process that requires real recovery time.

Let that sink in for a moment. You now understand more about the biology of your own condition than most people will ever learn. That understanding is the foundation for everything that comes next. In the next chapter, we're going to get specific—because migraine doesn't just have one face. It has an entire dysfunctional family. Time to meet them all.

Chapter 2: The Migraine Multiverse

Know Thy Enemy

Alright, warrior, welcome to the next level of your training. You've met the Four Horsemen. You know the biology is real. Now things get complicated.

But now, things get complicated.

If you thought "migraine" was a single villain, I'm about to ruin your day. It isn't one monster; it's a whole dysfunctional family, and each member has its own personality, signature moves, and preferred methods of making your life a living hell.

Why does this matter? Because you can't fight an enemy you can't identify. You wouldn't use a squirt gun in a sword fight, and you wouldn't bring a knife to a battle against a fire-breathing dragon. Knowing which specific demon you're dealing with is the first step toward finding the right weapons, building a targeted defense, and finally getting the upper hand.

Is your migraine the flashy Drama Queen that announces its arrival with a psychedelic light show? Or is it the Silent Ninja that ambushes you with zero warning? Is it the Relentless Roommate who decides to stick around for half the month? Or, and this is a big one, is it an imposter? A copycat condition like Occipital or Trigeminal Neuralgia that masquerades as a migraine but requires a completely different battle plan?

This chapter is your field guide to this multiverse of pain. It's your Pokédex of neurological nightmares. We're going to meet the whole rogue's gallery so you can look at your symptoms and say, "Aha! I know you, you son of a bitch."

To make this easy---because let's be honest, brain fog is real---we're going to start with a cheat sheet. This is your quick-and-dirty diagnostic tool.

What type of migraine do you have today?

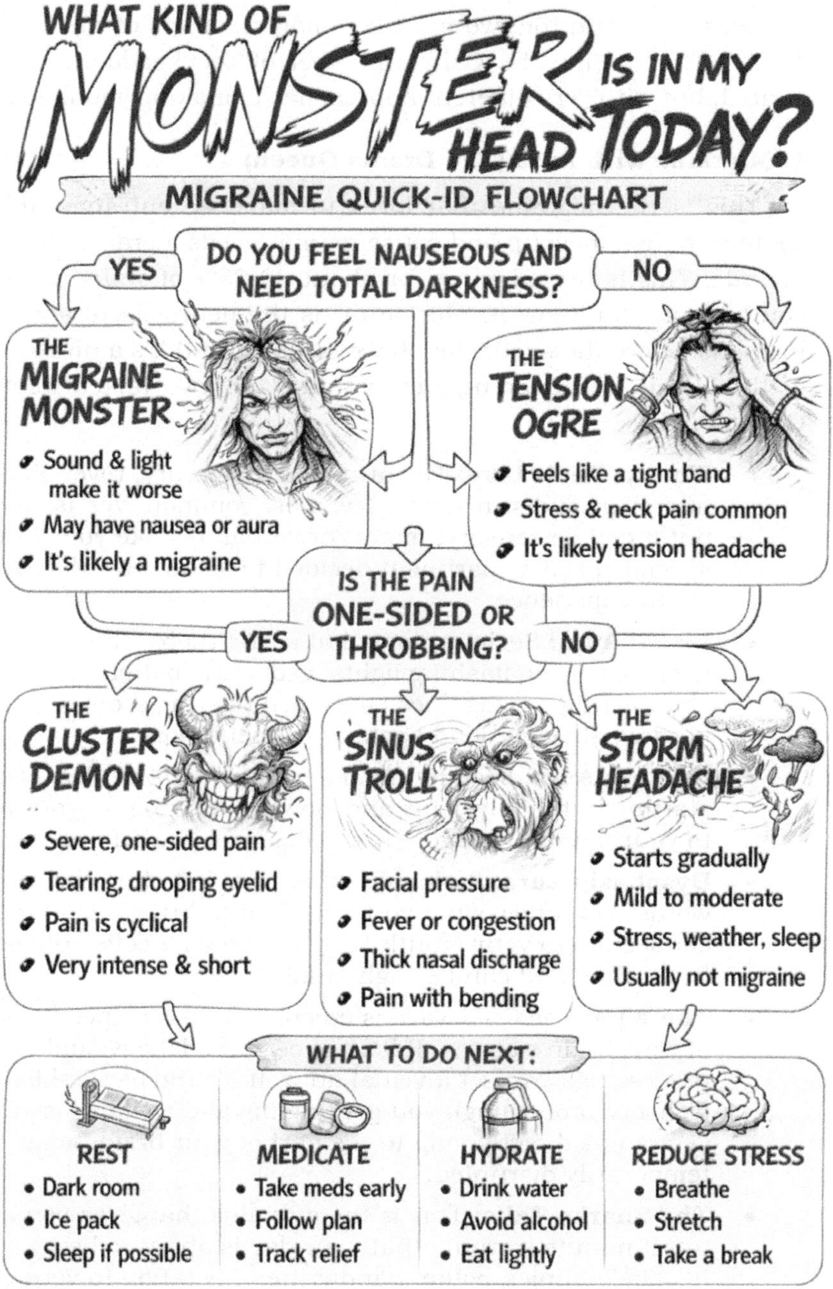

Image made with the help of AI.

The Main Players: The Two Faces of Classic Migraine

Let's start with the two most common members of the migraine family. They're like the Cain and Abel of the headache world---related, but with very different approaches to making you miserable.

1. Migraine with Aura (The Drama Queen)

This is the migraine that loves to make an entrance. It's not content to just show up and cause pain; it needs a grand, theatrical prelude. This is the migraine for about 20-25% of sufferers, and if you have it, you know it. The "aura" is the neurological show that happens before the headache phase kicks in, and it's a direct result of that Cortical Spreading Depression (CSD) we talked about in Chapter 1.

- **What It Feels Like:** The aura is a temporary, reversible neurological disturbance. The most common type is visual, but it can be sensory, motor, or verbal. It's like your brain's special effects department decided to go on a bender. You might experience:
- **Visual Aura:** Seeing things that aren't there. This can be positive (seeing flashing lights, geometric patterns, or shimmering zig-zag lines called scintillating scotoma) or negative (having blind spots or tunnel vision).
- **Sensory Aura:** Feeling tingling or pins-and-needles, often starting in the fingertips and slowly marching up your arm to your face and tongue. It can also feel like numbness.
- **Dysphasic Aura:** Suddenly being unable to find the right words. You know what you want to say, but your brain's connection to your mouth seems to be on a coffee break. It's frustrating and can be frightening.
- **The Why:** The CSD wave is creeping across a specific part of your brain's cortex. If it's the occipital lobe (visual processing), you get a visual aura. If it's the parietal lobe (sensory processing), you get tingling and numbness. The symptoms directly map to the part of your brain being temporarily disrupted.
- **The Snarky Take:** This is the migraine that gives you a 20-to-60-minute warning that your day is about to be ruined. It's like getting a polite, handwritten invitation to your own personal hell. Thanks, I guess?

2. Migraine without Aura (The Silent Ninja)

This is the most common form of migraine, affecting the vast majority of sufferers. This one skips the theatrics. There's no warning light show, no preview of the coming agony. It just... strikes. Like a ninja in the night, it appears suddenly and with ruthless efficiency, leaving you blindsided and reeling.

- What It Feels Like: All of the pain, none of the prelude. You might get some prodrome symptoms hours or a day before (like yawning or neck stiffness), but you don't get that immediate, "uh-oh, here it comes" aura. The attack phase begins with the full force of its symptoms:
- Intense, throbbing, one-sided head pain.
- Severe nausea and sometimes vomiting.
- Extreme sensitivity to light, sound, and smells.
- The overwhelming desire to crawl into a dark, silent hole and not emerge for three days.
- The Why: Your brain still goes through the same underlying process of neuronal hyper-excitability and chemical floods (hello, CGRP!), but for reasons scientists don't fully understand, it doesn't produce the perceptible wave of CSD that causes aura symptoms. It's all happening behind the scenes, until the pain makes its grand, unannounced entrance.
- The Snarky Take: This is the migraine with no manners. It doesn't even have the decency to call before it shows up to trash your house. Rude.

SIDEBAR SHOWDOWN: Migraine vs. Cluster Headache

People often confuse these two, but they are vastly different beasts. Think of it as a heavyweight boxer versus a knife-wielding assassin.

The Frequent Flyers: The Ones That Keep Coming Back

These are the migraine variants that aren't defined by their symptoms alone, but by their timing, persistence, and unique triggers. They're the ones that integrate themselves into the very rhythm of your life.

1. Chronic Migraine (The Relentless Roommate)

Imagine your average migraine, but instead of visiting for a day or two and then leaving, it decides to move in, put its feet on your coffee table, and never, ever leave. That's chronic migraine. The official definition is experiencing a headache on 15 or more days per month for at least three months, with at least 8 of those days meeting the criteria for migraine.

- What It Feels Like: A relentless, grinding state of near-constant head pain. On "good" days, it might just be a background tension-type headache. On bad days, it's a full-blown migraine attack. You live in a perpetual state of waiting for the other shoe to drop, because it usually already has. It's exhausting, demoralizing, and can lead to a significant decline in quality of life.
- The Why: Chronic migraine is often a progression from episodic migraine. It's like your brain's pain pathways have become so used to being activated that they get stuck in the "on" position. The threshold for triggering an attack drops lower and lower. Medication overuse is a common contributing factor, leading to a vicious cycle of rebound headaches that fuel the chronification.
- The Snarky Take: This is the clingy ex of migraines. It just can't take a hint, and now it's sleeping on your couch and using your toothbrush.

2. Vestibular Migraine (The Dizzy Spells)

This is the migraine that messes with your sense of reality. For people with vestibular migraine, the main event isn't always pain---it's vertigo and dizziness. The world starts to spin, tilt, or sway, as if you're drunk on a boat in the middle of a hurricane.

- What It Feels Like: The symptoms can be terrifying and disorienting. They can last for seconds, minutes, or even days, and they don't always come with a headache.

Spontaneous Vertigo: The room suddenly starts spinning for no reason.

Positional Vertigo: The spinning is triggered by changing your head position.

Disequilibrium: A constant feeling of being off-balance or unsteady on your feet.

Motion Sickness: Extreme sensitivity to any kind of motion, whether in a car or just watching a fast-paced movie.

- The Why: This migraine variant targets the vestibular system---the intricate network in your inner ear and brainstem that controls your balance and spatial orientation. The same neurological chaos that causes pain in a classic migraine instead causes a misfiring of the signals that tell your brain where your body is in space.
- The Snarky Take: This is the migraine that thinks gravity is a fun suggestion, not a law of physics. It turns your life into a carnival funhouse, except there's no fun and you can't get off the ride.

3. Menstrual Migraine (The Monthly Menace)

For many people who menstruate, there's a dreaded, predictable pattern: when their period is about to start, a migraine comes knocking. This isn't a coincidence; it's a direct result of hormonal warfare.

- What It Feels Like: These attacks are often more severe, last longer, and are more resistant to treatment than migraines at other times of the month. They typically occur in the two days leading up to the start of menstruation and the first three days of it.
- The Why: It's all about the estrogen drop. In the late luteal phase of the menstrual cycle, right before your period begins, there's a sharp decline in estrogen levels. This sudden hormonal plunge is believed to make the brain more susceptible to migraine triggers. It lowers your migraine threshold, so things that might not have bothered you a week earlier can now set off a catastrophic attack.
- The Snarky Take: It's your body's monthly subscription service for misery. As if cramps, bloating, and mood swings weren't enough, it throws in a skull-splitting headache for free. What a bargain.

The Rare & Terrifying: The Heavyweights of the Multiverse

Now we venture into the territory of the rare, the strange, and the frankly terrifying. These migraine variants are less common, but they are critically important to know about because their symptoms can be alarming and often mimic other serious medical emergencies. If you suspect you have one of these, the first step is always to seek immediate medical evaluation to rule out anything more sinister.

1. Hemiplegic Migraine (The Stroke Impostor)

This is, without a doubt, one of the most frightening members of the migraine family. The word "hemiplegic" means paralysis on one side of the body. That's right. This migraine variant has the audacious cruelty to perfectly mimic the symptoms of a stroke.

- What It Feels Like: A hemiplegic migraine attack includes the typical migraine aura, but with a terrifying addition: temporary, one-sided motor weakness or paralysis. This isn't just a bit of tingling; it's a noticeable loss of motor control. Symptoms can include:
- Weakness on one side of the body, ranging from mild clumsiness to full paralysis of an arm and leg.
- Slurred speech or difficulty finding words (aphasia).
- Numbness and tingling that spreads over one side of the body.
- Confusion, drowsiness, or even loss of consciousness in severe cases.
- These symptoms are then typically followed by a severe, throbbing headache, although sometimes the headache is mild or absent.
- The Why: This isn't your standard-issue CSD. Hemiplegic migraine is strongly linked to specific genetic mutations in genes that control ion channels in the brain (like CACNA1A, ATP1A2, and SCN1A). These faulty channels disrupt the normal electrical signaling between neurons, leading to the profound and widespread neurological symptoms. There are two types: Familial Hemiplegic Migraine (FHM), which runs in families, and Sporadic Hemiplegic Migraine (SHM), for those of us who just won the world's worst genetic lottery.
- The Snarky (but Serious) Take: This is the migraine that's a pathological method actor, giving a frighteningly convincing performance of a stroke. If you ever experience symptoms like this, especially for the first time, don't play guessing games. Go to the emergency room. Let the doctors be the ones to tell you, "Congratulations, it's not a stroke, just the most terrifying migraine known to science."

2. Retinal Migraine (The One-Eyed Terror)

While a standard visual aura affects both eyes (because it originates in the brain's visual cortex), a retinal migraine is different. It's an eye problem, not just a brain problem, and it involves temporary vision loss in one single eye.

- What It Feels Like: Sufferers describe a range of frightening visual symptoms that occur in only one eye and typically last for less than an hour:
- Scintillations (seeing twinkling or flashing lights).
- Scotoma (areas of decreased or lost vision, like a blind spot that gets larger).
- Temporary, partial, or complete blindness in that one eye.
- This visual disturbance is usually followed by or occurs during a typical migraine headache.
- The Why: Unlike a typical aura, the problem here is thought to be with the blood vessels that supply the retina---the light-sensitive layer at the back of the eye. It's believed that a spasm or reduced blood flow in the retinal artery causes the temporary vision loss.
- The Snarky Take: This is the migraine that decides to play a magic trick on you. "Now you see... now you don't!" It's not amusing, and it's another one that warrants a serious conversation with a specialist (like an ophthalmologist and a neurologist) to make sure nothing else sinister is going on with your eye.

SIDEBAR SHOWDOWN: Tension Headache vs. Occipital Neuralgia

Many people assume any pain in the head that isn't a full-blown migraine must be a tension headache. Wrong. Meet Occipital Neuralgia, the imposter that lives in your neck.

The Neck & Nerve Connection: The Hidden Culprits

Alright, let's talk about the impostors. These are the conditions that aren't technically migraines but are so often confused with them that they deserve their own special section in this book. For countless sufferers, the answer to their chronic head pain doesn't lie entirely within the brain itself but in the complex and often-abused network of nerves in their neck and face. If you've tried every migraine treatment under the sun with no relief, this section is for you.

1. Occipital Neuralgia (ON): The Neck's Revenge

This is one of the most under-diagnosed and misunderstood causes of head pain. Occipital Neuralgia isn't a primary headache disorder like migraine; it's a nerve condition. Specifically, it's caused by the irritation or compression of the occipital nerves. These nerves run from the top of your spinal cord, up through the muscles at the back of your neck, and into your scalp, providing sensation to the back and top of your head. When these nerves are unhappy, they let you know. Loudly.

- What It Feels Like (Hint: Not Like a Migraine): The defining feature of ON is the quality of the pain. Forget the deep, throbbing pulse of a migraine. ON pain is characteristically:

Sharp, shooting, and zapping. Many describe it as a brief, intense electric shock that runs up the back of their head.

Stabbing or piercing. It can feel like you're being jabbed with an ice pick.

- The pain follows the path of the nerve, usually starting in the upper neck or at the base of the skull and shooting upwards.
- Between the sharp attacks, you might have a persistent, aching, or burning sensation.
- Your scalp often becomes incredibly tender. Even brushing your hair or resting your head on a pillow can be excruciating.
- The Why: What makes the occipital nerves so angry? Usually, it's because they're being pinched, compressed, or inflamed. Common causes include:
- Tight neck muscles: Years of poor posture (hello, "tech neck") can cause the muscles at the base of your skull to tighten and entrap the nerves.

Injury: Trauma to the back of the head, like from whiplash in a car accident.

- Underlying Conditions: Osteoarthritis in the cervical spine or other degenerative disc diseases can put pressure on the nerves.
- Sometimes, there's no clear cause, which is just as frustrating.
- The Great Overlap (Why It's So Confusing): If it's so different, why is it confused with migraine? Because the pain can be severe, unilateral, and debilitating. Even more confusingly, the intense, painful signals from an ON flare-

up can actually trigger a true migraine in someone who is already susceptible. Your brain interprets the overwhelming nerve pain from your neck as a threat, and in response, it kicks off the whole Four Horsemen cascade. You end up with a horrific hybrid attack: the zapping, stabbing pain of ON combined with the nausea, light sensitivity, and throbbing misery of a migraine. This is why a specialist diagnosis is absolutely essential.

📖 Ken's Corner: The First Time My Face Went Numb — and What It Actually Meant

I want to tell you about a moment that completely changed how I understood my own condition. If neck involvement plays any role in your head pain, something similar may have happened to you too—and if it has, it probably scared the hell out of you.

For me, it happened on July 21st, 2021, during the COVID lockdown. I was sitting at my desk at home working when a sudden bolt of pain hit the top right side of my head. Not a normal headache. It felt like someone had driven an ice pick straight into my skull. Within seconds something even stranger happened. My upper arms and shoulders stopped working. My forearms and hands still functioned, but I couldn't lift my arms or move my shoulders. When I tried to stand, I could only shuffle my feet. My speech was slurred, the left side of my face stopped moving, and my thinking felt foggy and slow.

In that moment I was absolutely certain I was having a stroke. I tried to dial 911, but here's the surreal part: I couldn't figure out how to do it. My brain simply wouldn't cooperate. The last person I had spoken to earlier that day was my wife, so I called her instead. She immediately realized something was very wrong. She called 911 for me and raced back to the house. The ambulance arrived quickly. My wife reached the street just as they were pulling away and followed the ambulance to the hospital on her motorcycle.

At the ER the staff moved fast because everyone assumed the same thing I did—stroke. They ran neurological exams, blood work, and imaging. The blood work looked normal, which confused everyone. Then they rushed me into an MRI. While I was lying inside the scanner, something strange began to happen. The paralysis started fading. My facial numbness began to lift, and I slowly regained movement in my shoulders and arms. At first, I didn't say anything because I hadn't realized the change was happening until it was already underway.

About an hour later the doctors came back with the results. It wasn't a stroke. It was a **hemiplegic migraine**, a rare type of migraine that can mimic stroke symptoms almost perfectly. For the next four and a half years, I got used to having two to three hemiplegic migraines a week, even while at work.

That was my formal reintroduction to the migraine world. I had experienced migraines as a teenager, but they had mostly disappeared by the time I reached my twenties. Suddenly they were back—and this time they had escalated into something far more dramatic.

Over the following months and years, I began noticing a strange pattern. Whenever I helped my wife move heavy equipment for her business, worked on our house, lifted furniture, or worked on our cars—activities that involved bending, lifting, and awkward neck positions—the same symptoms would return. Usually about an hour later, the left side of my face would go numb. Not tingling. Numb. The left half of my upper lip would lose sensation, and a patch of scalp behind and above my left ear would feel strangely deadened.

The facial numbness was not the only pattern that followed physical strain. Over time I also developed hyperacusis—an extreme sensitivity to sound that went far beyond normal discomfort. Loud or sudden noise could trigger projectile vomiting, loss of consciousness, and a complete neurological shutdown. It happened at work when I stepped off an elevator into a noisy floor and collapsed, carried away by coworkers. It happened in a doctor's waiting room when raised voices and children screaming overwhelmed my system in seconds. Like the facial numbness, it was terrifying at first—and like the facial numbness, it eventually revealed itself as part of the same reproducible pattern.

Every time my neck was heavily loaded—whether from helping my wife haul equipment, working under a car, or even spending long hours hunched at my desk producing corporate training videos—the same cascade followed. The numbness, the sound sensitivity, the neurological fog. It was not random. It was reproducible. And that reproducibility was the clue that changed everything.

That realization eventually led me to a question that took years to answer: how could a neck problem cause numbness in the face and severe hyperacusis?

On the surface, it shouldn't. The nerves in your neck don't directly supply sensation to your face. Facial sensation is controlled by the trigeminal nerve, a cranial nerve that originates in the brainstem, not the cervical spine. So how could disc degeneration, bone spurs, and spinal stenosis at levels like C2 or C3 cause facial symptoms?

The answer lies in a structure in the brainstem called the **trigeminocervical nucleus**. This region acts as a shared processing center where upper cervical nerve fibers (C1 through C3) and trigeminal sensory fibers converge. They feed into the same neurological circuitry. When chronic irritation in the upper cervical spine—caused by things like facet arthritis, bone spurs, or narrowing around the nerve openings—keeps those cervical nerves firing repeatedly, the brainstem's processing center becomes overloaded. Because trigeminal fibers share that same neural "real estate," the brain can misinterpret where the signal originated.

In other words, the source of my facial numbness was not a problem in my brain or face. The signal was originating in my cervical spine, but my brain's shared processing center could not distinguish it from a trigeminal event—so it interpreted the pain as coming from my face.

This neurological convergence also explains why cervicogenic headaches can feel almost identical to classic migraines. The same brainstem pathways process both signals. My doctors weren't wrong to treat me for migraines—they simply didn't yet know what was driving the signal upstream.

There was another clue I ignored for years. On the right side of my scalp I had a small hypersensitive patch of skin that felt slightly raised and extremely tender. Touching it produced a sharp, burning pain that shot across my scalp. At the time I assumed it was just another strange symptom of my situation. In reality, it was a sensitized branch of the **greater occipital nerve**, a classic sign of chronic occipital neuralgia.

I had received nerve ablations several times targeting the C2 areas on both sides, and while each round helped reduce the intensity of my daily migraines for five to six months, the migraines themselves never stopped. Not once in four and a half years. They would drop from a level seven through ten down to a level two through four—which, in hindsight, should have been yet another clue that my pain was being driven by a structural problem in the neck, not a purely neurochemical one.

Most people who have typical migraines experience days, weeks, or even months of remission between attacks. Mine never remitted. Twenty-four hours a day for four and a half years, I was in some degree of pain. In hindsight, that single fact was the most telling breadcrumb of all—pointing straight to the structural source of the problem. The clues were there the entire time. We just weren't reading them correctly.

If any part of this story sounds familiar to you—the facial numbness, the scalp tenderness, the symptoms that appear after heavy lifting or neck strain and improve when you lie flat on your back with no pillow—it may be worth discussing **cervicogenic headache and occipital neuralgia** with your physician. And if that possibility resonates with your experience, the next section was written specifically for you.

2. Trigeminal Neuralgia (TN): The Face's Fury

If Occipital Neuralgia is the neck's revenge, Trigeminal Neuralgia is a full-scale assault on your face. Often called the "suicide disease" because of the sheer intensity of the pain, TN is widely considered to be one of the most painful conditions known to medicine. It's a disorder of the trigeminal nerve---yes, the same nerve that's a key player in migraine---but the mechanism and symptoms are brutally different.

What It Feels Like: The pain of TN is legendary in its cruelty. It's not an ache or a throb. It is:

An intense, stabbing, electric shock-like pain in the face. It's almost always unilateral.

- The attacks are typically very brief, lasting from a few seconds to a couple of minutes, but they can occur in rapid, repetitive succession.
- The pain is confined to the areas supplied by the trigeminal nerve: the lower jaw, the cheek, the upper jaw, and sometimes the area around the eye and forehead.

- The Triggers (The Defining Feature): This is what truly separates TN. The pain is often triggered by the most mundane, gentle stimuli. Things that should never, ever cause pain suddenly become triggers for excruciating agony:
- Touching your face lightly
- Brushing your teeth
- Shaving or applying makeup
- A gentle breeze on your skin
- Smiling, talking, or chewing
- The Why: The most common cause of TN is a blood vessel (usually an artery) pressing on the trigeminal nerve at the point where it exits the brainstem. This constant pulsation from the vessel wears away the protective sheath (myelin) around the nerve, causing it to send chaotic, short-circuiting pain signals at the slightest touch.
- The Great Overlap: While the pain itself is distinct, the involvement of the trigeminal nerve creates confusion. The nerve becomes so sensitized from TN that it can, like ON, trigger a secondary migraine attack. People with pre-existing migraines might also develop TN, leading to a complex and overlapping pain profile that requires careful diagnosis by a neurologist or facial pain specialist.

☐ Clinical Note: When "Migraines" Are Something Else Entirely

For physicians, neurologists, nurse practitioners, physician assistants, and any clinician who treats patients with chronic headache.

The patient in front of you may have been treated for primary migraine for years. Their chart may say "chronic migraine" or "migraine without aura." Their previous providers were not wrong to try migraine-specific treatments. But if that patient has exhausted multiple preventive and acute therapies with incomplete or frustrating results, consider whether the primary driver of their pain is actually structural -- not neurochemical.

The clinical profile worth pausing on: head and/or neck pain that is worsened by neck movement or specific postures, reduced cervical range of motion, unilateral scalp tenderness along the greater occipital nerve distribution, partial but not complete response to occipital nerve blocks, and symptoms that are reliably reproduced by physical loading of the cervical spine (bending, lifting, sustained postures).

When the patient also has documented cervical degenerative disease -- facet arthropathy, disc-osteophyte complexes, foraminal narrowing -- the convergence of structural findings and clinical presentation deserves direct attention.

Cervicogenic headache and Occipital Neuralgia are not rare. They are underdiagnosed, particularly in patients who also carry a primary migraine diagnosis -- because they can coexist, and because the phenotypic overlap is substantial.

The trigeminocervical convergence means that upper cervical irritation (C1-C3) produces pain that is centrally processed identically to trigeminal-mediated migraine pain. Patients are not exaggerating. Their brain genuinely cannot distinguish the source.

A targeted diagnostic approach -- cervical imaging if not recently obtained, diagnostic medial branch blocks at the symptomatic levels, and explicit clinical examination of the upper cervical spine -- can be profoundly clarifying. And for patients whose "migraine" resolves or dramatically improves following a diagnostic cervical injection, that response is the diagnosis.

Patients who have done their own research, including AI-assisted review of their imaging reports, may arrive at your office with specific questions about cervicogenic mechanisms and structural contributors.

They deserve to have those questions engaged with seriously. They are not seeking to direct their own treatment; they are trying to be useful partners in a diagnostic process that has frustrated them for years.

— *Clinical content reviewed by* ***Elliott James, APRN, MSN, CMRD***

Chapter Two Conclusion: Why Knowing Your Enemy Is Half the Battle

And there you have it---a whirlwind tour of the Migraine Multiverse. We've met the common players, the frequent flyers, the rare and terrifying assassins, and the insidious impostors. If your head is spinning (and not from a vestibular migraine, hopefully), that's okay.

The purpose of this chapter isn't for you to self-diagnose. It's to arm you with knowledge. It's to give you the language and understanding to look at your own experience and start connecting the dots. Does your "migraine" always start with a zapping pain in your neck? Maybe it's time to ask a doctor about Occipital Neuralgia. Do you get debilitating dizzy spells without a headache? That sounds like a conversation about Vestibular Migraine.

This is what changes the game. When you go to your doctor, you can now say, "I think I might have Migraine with Aura," or "My symptoms seem to align more with Occipital Neuralgia. Could we explore that?" This is how you advocate for yourself. This is how you get the right diagnosis and, ultimately, the right treatment.

Now that you know who the enemy is---or at least have a list of prime suspects---it's time to learn their tactics. In the next section, PART II: ANTICIPATE, we're going to become migraine psychics. We'll learn how to decode the signals, track the triggers, and see an attack coming before it has a chance to strike. Understanding the enemy is half the battle; foresight is the other half. Let's learn to see the future.

Chapter 3: Anatomy of an Attack

The Four-Act Tragedy

If you've ever felt like your migraines come out of nowhere, ambushing you with the subtlety of a flashbang grenade in a library, you're probably wrong. And I say that with love.

Migraines are rarely a surprise attack. They follow a script—a predictable, four-act structure that can span hours or even days. The problem is, no one ever gave you the playbill.

This chapter is your copy of the script.

Our mission is to dissect this four-act tragedy so you can learn to recognize the subtle foreshadowing in Act I, brace for the rising action in Act II, and maybe, just maybe, intervene before the catastrophe of Act III. When you know the script, you stop being a victim of the play and start becoming its director. You can see what's coming and change the ending.

So, grab your popcorn (unless that's a trigger), because the show is about to begin.

This is the most misunderstood and frequently missed phase of a migraine attack. The prodrome is the weird, subtle, and deeply personal set of clues your body gives you hours, or even a full day or two, before the headache kicks in. It's your brain's passive-aggressive way of whispering, "I'm about to ruin you. Good luck."

Many people dismiss these symptoms as just a weird off-day. They'll say, "I don't know why, I just feel strange today," or "I was so tired yesterday for no reason." Spoiler alert: there was a reason. Your brain was already starting the engine for the migraine express.

Recognizing your personal prodrome symptoms is your superpower. This is your golden window of opportunity to intervene. It's the point where you might be able to blunt the coming attack or, on a truly glorious day, stop it in its tracks entirely.

The migraine timeline:

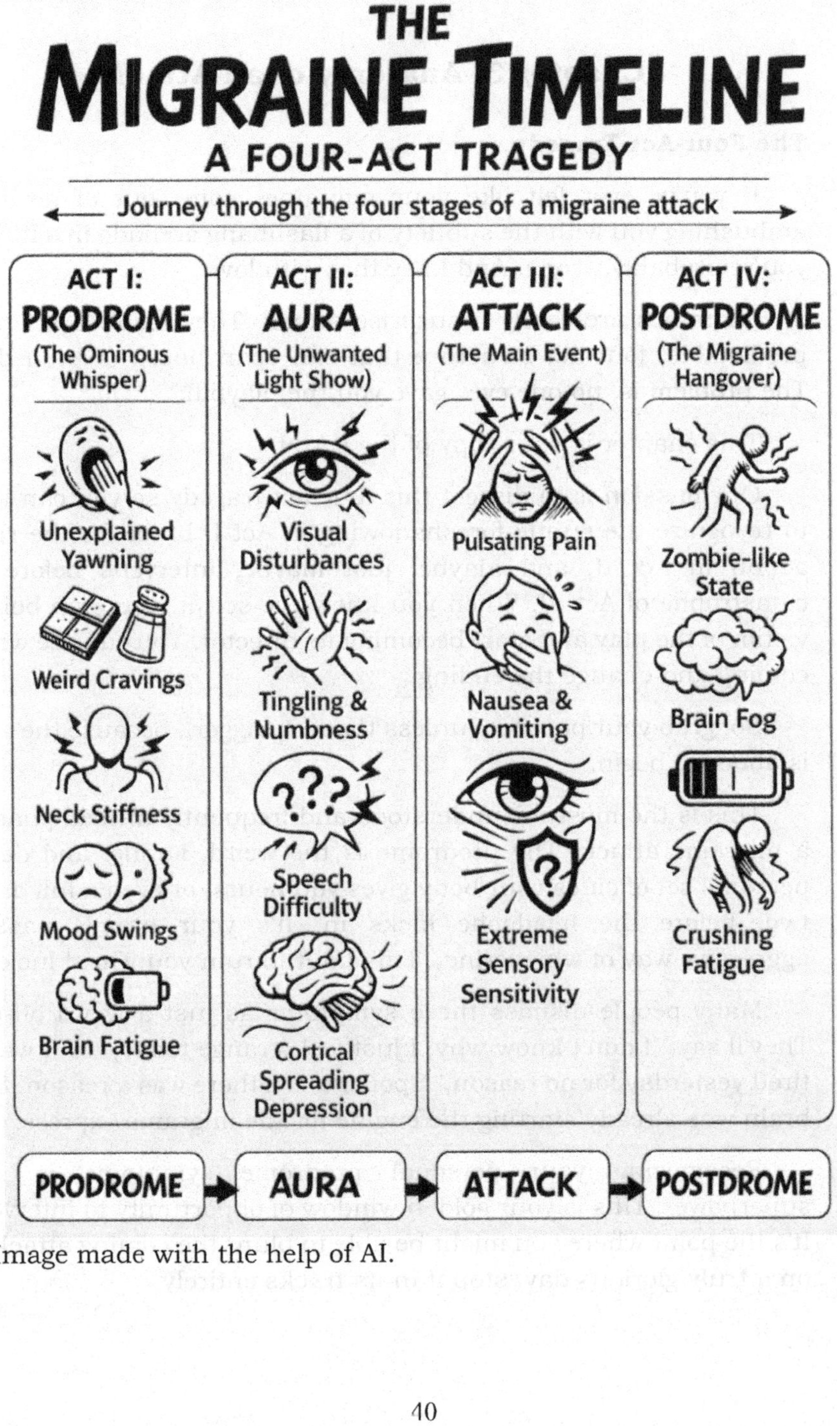

Image made with the help of AI.

Here are the most common characters in the prodrome cast:

- Unexplained Fatigue & Yawning: This isn't your typical "I need a coffee" tiredness. This is a sudden, profound wave of exhaustion that seems to come from nowhere. You might find yourself yawning uncontrollably, even if you got a full night's sleep. This is thought to be linked to the hypothalamus, the part of your brain that acts as a master regulator for sleep and energy, starting to go on the fritz.
- Mood Swings: Do you suddenly feel irritable and want to snap at everyone? Or, conversely, do you feel strangely euphoric, energetic, and giddy for no reason? These abrupt shifts in mood are classic prodrome symptoms, also tied to the dysregulation of brain chemicals like dopamine and serotonin. If you suddenly feel like you could either conquer the world or burn it to the ground, a migraine might be brewing.
- Neck Stiffness: This is a big one that many people mistake for the cause of their headache, when it's often the symptom of a coming migraine. You might feel a dull ache or stiffness in your neck and shoulders. This is a signal from the brainstem and the trigeminal nerve pathways getting fired up. Your neck isn't causing the migraine; the brewing migraine is causing your neck to hurt.
- Weird Food Cravings: Suddenly have an insatiable urge for something specific, often salty or sweet? It's not just a random whim. Your hypothalamus is at it again, messing with your appetite regulation. The cruel irony is that the very food you crave (like chocolate) might also be a trigger for you, making it a delicious but treacherous trap.
- Increased Urination: If you find yourself running to the bathroom more often than usual without having increased your fluid intake, this can be another sneaky prodrome sign. Once again, blame the hypothalamus, which helps regulate your body's fluid balance.
- Heightened Sensitivities: Long before the full-blown sensory assault of the attack phase, you might notice subtle sensitivities. Lights might seem a little too bright, or sounds might be just a bit more annoying than usual. This is your brain's volume knob slowly being turned up to eleven.

Learning to spot these whispers is the first step to hijacking the script. If you start to notice a personal pattern---"Every time I get that weird neck stiffness and crave potato chips, I get a migraine the next day"---you've just found the keys to the kingdom.

Act II: The Aura (The Unwanted Light Show)

Welcome to the second act, the part of the show that only about a quarter of migraine sufferers get to experience. If you're one of them, you know that the aura is your brain's personal, and entirely unwanted, psychedelic art exhibit. It's the final, flashing, neon warning sign before the main event.

The aura is a series of temporary neurological symptoms that typically last from five minutes to an hour. And just to be clear, it's not a hallucination. It's a real, measurable electrical event in your brain. Remember Cortical Spreading Depression (CSD) from Chapter 1? This is its time to shine. The CSD is that slow wave of electrical hyper-activity followed by inactivity, and as it crawls across the surface of your brain, it disrupts the normal function of whatever area it touches. The symptoms you experience directly correspond to the path that wave takes.

Here are the most common types of aura:

- Visual Aura (The Brain's Glitchy Screensaver): This is the most famous type. It happens when the CSD wave moves across your visual cortex. It can manifest in a few ways:
- Scintillating Scotoma: This is the classic. It often starts as a small spot of shimmering, flickering, or jagged zig-zagging light near the center of your vision. It then slowly expands and drifts across your visual field over the course of 20-30 minutes, often leaving a blind spot in its wake. It can look like a shimmering, C-shaped kaleidoscope of broken glass.
- Blind Spots (Negative Scotoma): You might experience holes in your vision, like parts of the world have just been deleted.

Tunnel Vision: Your peripheral vision might close in, making it feel like you're looking through a tube.

- Sensory Aura (The March of the Tingles): This happens when the CSD wave hits your sensory cortex. It typically starts as a pins-and-needles sensation in your fingertips on one side of your body. Over several minutes, it will slowly "march" up your arm, sometimes to your face, lips, and tongue. It can also manifest as numbness, where it feels like a part of your body has gone to sleep.

- Dysphasic Aura (The Word Salad Catastrophe): This is when the CSD wave passes over your brain's language centers. It's a deeply unsettling experience where you suddenly find yourself unable to articulate your thoughts. You might struggle to find the right words, use the wrong words, or speak in jumbled, nonsensical sentences. You know what you want to say, but the connection is temporarily broken.

The aura phase, while often frightening, is the most definitive "Code Red" warning you will ever get. The moment it starts, the clock is ticking. This is your last chance to deploy your acute attack plan (which we'll cover in Chapter 6) before the pain takes over.

Act III: The Attack (The Main Event)

If the prodrome was the whisper and the aura was the flashing warning light, the attack phase is the full-blown, category-five hurricane making landfall directly on your skull. This is the part of the migraine that gets all the press, the part that has you curled in a fetal position, bargaining with deities you don't believe in.

This is where the Four Horsemen from Chapter 1 are in full gallop. The CGRP is flooding your system, the blood vessels are throwing their throbbing rave, and neuro-inflammation is setting everything on fire. The result is a multi-sensory experience of pure, unadulterated suck.

Let's break down the headliners of this terrible show:

The Pain: This isn't just pain; it's an event. Migraine pain has a distinct personality, and it's a real jerk.

- Quality: It's almost always throbbing or pulsating. This is the work of the Vascular Mayhem horseman. Your inflamed, dilated blood vessels are literally throbbing in time with your heartbeat, sending waves of agony through your head.
- Location: It's typically unilateral, meaning it camps out on one side of your head. It can be behind your eye, in your temple, or across one entire hemisphere of your brain. For extra fun, it can sometimes switch sides during an attack or even become bilateral.

- Intensity: It ranges from moderate to severe, but "severe" in the migraine world means "questioning the will to live." It's a pain so profound it can feel like it has a physical weight.
- The Nausea (and its evil twin, Vomiting): As if the head-splitting pain weren't enough, your stomach decides to join the rebellion. The connection between your brain and your gut is a powerful one (the "gut-brain axis"), and during a migraine, this communication line goes haywire. Your brainstem, which houses the "vomit center," gets activated by the neurological chaos, leading to waves of nausea that can be just as debilitating as the pain itself. For many, this culminates in vomiting, which, in a moment of cruel relief, can sometimes temporarily lessen the headache intensity before it comes roaring back.
- The Sensory Assault (When the World Becomes the Enemy): During an attack, your brain loses its ability to filter sensory information. The gatekeepers that normally keep the world at a manageable volume are offline, and every sight, sound, and smell becomes an attack.
- Photophobia (Sensitivity to Light): This is the "vampire mode." Normal indoor lighting can feel like staring into the sun. Sunlight is a physical punishment. The light signals traveling from your eye to your brain are amplified, creating an experience of intense pain. This is why a dark, silent cave becomes your greatest ambition.
- Phonophobia & Hyperacusis (Sensitivity to Sound): Phonophobia is an aversion to sound; hyperacusis is when normal sounds are perceived as painfully, unbearably loud. The gentle hum of the refrigerator sounds like a jet engine. A normal conversation feels like being screamed at through a megaphone. The sound-processing centers in your brain are in overdrive, and every noise is an irritant.
- Osmophobia (Sensitivity to Smell): Smells you might normally enjoy, like coffee brewing or a scented candle, can become nauseating and trigger a worsening of the pain. Your olfactory system is on high alert, and it has decided that everything stinks.

This unholy trinity of pain, nausea, and sensory overload is the core of the attack phase. It can last anywhere from four hours to a brutal 72 hours (or longer, in the case of the dreaded status migrainosus). This isn't a phase you "power through." This is a phase you survive.

If you have cervical involvement in your headache picture, vestibular symptoms can sometimes appear during treatment — and they are usually temporary. For a full discussion of the cervical-vestibular connection, see the preventive strategies in Chapter 7.

Act IV: The Postdrome (The Migraine Hangover)

The throbbing has subsided. The nausea has passed. You've emerged from your cave, blinking in the tentatively-not-painful light. The war is over, right?

Wrong. Welcome to Act IV, the postdrome, more affectionately known as the Migraine Hangover.

This is the phase that family, friends, and employers almost never understand. They see the main attack is over and assume you should be back to 100%. But you feel like a zombie, a ghost, a human-shaped shell filled with brain fog and exhaustion. Your body might have survived the battle, but the battlefield is an absolute wreck, and the cleanup is going to take a while. The postdrome can linger for 24 to 48 hours after the headache is gone.

Here's what the hangover feels like:

- Crushing Fatigue: This is the most common postdrome symptom. It's not just being tired; it's a bone-deep, cellular exhaustion. Your brain and body have just expended a tremendous amount of energy fighting a multi-day neurological war. You've depleted your neurotransmitters and flooded your system with inflammatory chemicals. Of course you're exhausted.
- Brain Fog (or "Migraine Brain"): This is the cognitive price you pay. You might struggle with concentration, have difficulty finding words (again), feel mentally slow, or have trouble with your memory. Your brain is literally in recovery mode, trying to sweep up the chemical debris and reset its circuits. It's no wonder you can't remember why you walked into a room.
- Lingering Sensitivity: While not as extreme as during the attack, you might still find light and sound to be irritating. Your brain's volume knob is still turned up a bit too high.
- Muscle Aches and Neck Pain: The tension from enduring hours of intense pain often leaves your neck, shoulders, and back feeling sore and achy.

- Weird Moods: Some people feel depressed or irritable during the postdrome. Others experience a strange sense of mild euphoria or relief. It's your brain chemistry slowly trying to find its way back to baseline.

The postdrome is a legitimate and crucial part of the migraine attack. It is not laziness. It is not you being dramatic. It is your body's necessary recovery process. Honoring this phase with rest, hydration, and gentle self-care is essential for a full recovery. Pushing through it is a recipe for triggering the next attack.

❤️□ A Note to Your Inner Circle: What's Actually Happening, Phase by Phase

For the people who love someone with migraines -- the partners, parents, friends, and anyone else who has stood at the bedroom door wondering what to do and how to help.

The four-act structure you just read about isn't just an explanation for the person with migraines. It's a roadmap for you, too. Because each phase looks and feels different from the outside -- and what helps in one phase can actually make things worse in another.

Here's your quick-reference guide.

The most important thing to understand is this: the attack doesn't end when the headache ends. The postdrome is real, it is biological, and it is not an excuse to keep resting. When your person says they're still not right the day after an attack, they're telling you the truth. Their brain is still in cleanup mode. Give them the time they need without making them justify it.

You don't have to fix this. You just have to not make it worse -- and sometimes, that's everything.

Your Field Guide Tools: The Cheat Sheets

Knowledge is only power if you can use it. Here are two quick-reference tools to help you start recognizing the script of your own attacks and intervening like a pro. Snap a photo of these, print them out, stick them on your fridge---whatever it takes.

Cheat Sheet #1: The Prodrome Red-Flag Checklist

Think of this as your personal early-warning system. If you check three or more of these boxes in a 24-hour period for no other reason, a migraine might be on its way. It's time to initiate your personal "Code Yellow" protocol (hydrate, avoid triggers, get extra rest, and have your rescue meds ready).

My Personal Prodrome Flags:

- [ ] Unexplained, deep-seated fatigue
- [ ] Excessive, uncontrollable yawning
- [ ] Unexplained neck or shoulder stiffness
- [ ] Sudden mood shift (irritable, anxious, or weirdly happy)
- [ ] Specific food cravings (What are yours? Salty? Sweet? ____________)
- [ ] Increased sensitivity to light or sound
- [ ] Frequent urination
- [ ] Brain feels "fuzzy" or slow
- [ ] Feeling unusually cold or having chills
- [ ] Other personal clue: __________________

Cheat Sheet #2: Early Intervention Cue Cards

Use these as mental flashcards. When you feel the cue, perform the action. The faster you act, the better your chances.

CUE CARD #1 IF YOU FEEL: The weird, subtle "something's not right" feelings of PRODROME... THEN YOU:

HYDRATE: Drink a large glass of water, preferably with electrolytes.

- MEDITATE (on your meds): Assess if it's time for a pre-emptive dose of an NSAID or your rescue medication (as discussed with your doctor).

DEFEND: Avoid your known triggers like the plague. Cancel that happy hour. Skip the intense workout.

REST: Prioritize an early night and gentle activity.

CUE CARD #2 IF YOU SEE/FEEL: The unmistakable visual or sensory symptoms of AURA... THEN YOU:

ACT NOW: Take your fast-acting rescue medication immediately. This is your best and last chance to stop the pain phase.

FIND SAFE HARBOR: Stop what you're doing (especially driving). Get to a safe, dark, quiet place.

ALERT YOUR CREW: Let a partner, friend, or coworker know what's happening.

CUE CARD #3 IF YOU FEEL: The first throb or wave of nausea from the ATTACK phase... THEN YOU:

DEPLOY THE TOOLKIT: If you haven't already, take your meds, grab your ice packs, and retreat to your migraine cave.

CANCEL EVERYTHING: This is not the time to be a hero. Send the "I'm bailing" text without guilt.

GO DARK: Eliminate all light and sound. Your only job now is to rest and survive.

Conclusion: You Now Have the Script. Use It.

And... scene.

You've just walked through the entire four-act tragedy of a migraine attack, from the first ominous whisper to the zombie-like hangover. It's a lot to take in, but now you have something most migraine sufferers never get: the script. You know the characters, you know the cues, and you know how the plot unfolds.

So, what's the actionable advice? What do you do with this newfound power?

You become a detective of your own body. Starting today, pay attention. When you feel "off," pull out that Prodrome Checklist. When you feel that familiar ache in your neck, don't just dismiss it. Ask yourself: Is this a sign? Keep your diary, learn your personal cues, and get ruthlessly good at recognizing Act I. The single most effective way to change the outcome of this play is to intervene before the curtain rises on Act III.

You now understand that your post-migraine fatigue isn't laziness---it's a biological recovery process. So, give yourself permission to rest. Defend that time fiercely. Explain it to your loved ones using the "brain on fire" analogy if you have to. Or hand them the phase guide above and let it do the explaining for you.

You are the expert on your own experience. By understanding the anatomy of your attacks, you can communicate more effectively with your doctors, advocate for yourself more confidently, and, most importantly, be kinder to yourself through the process.

Now that we know the what and the when of an attack, it's time to figure out the why. Why did the show start in the first place? What clumsy stagehand tripped over the power cord and kicked this whole thing off? That, my friend, is the world of triggers, and it's where we're headed next. Welcome to Part II: ANTICIPATE.

Chapter 4: The Trigger Minefield

Dodging the Dominoes

Welcome to Part II, where we move from understanding the enemy to anticipating its every move. We're going to learn how to decode the signals your body is sending and see an attack coming before it strikes. No crystal ball required—just data and a willingness to become the Sherlock Holmes of your own nervous system.

We begin this journey by stepping into the most treacherous territory of all: the Trigger Minefield.

If you're a migraine warrior, you've likely been conditioned to fear triggers. They are the boogeymen of our world---the flashing lights, the glass of red wine, the impending storm front, the very existence of your loud-chewing coworker. We're taught to identify them and avoid them at all costs, to the point where life can shrink until it fits inside a dark, quiet, scent-free, joy-free box.

But here's what most trigger guides get wrong: triggers are not all-powerful. They are data points, clues, and most importantly, they are rarely strong enough to act alone.

This is the most critical concept to grasp about triggers: a single trigger is rarely the culprit. A migraine attack is not usually the result of one thing. It's the result of a conspiracy. It's a perfectly aligned cascade of events, a series of unfortunate dominoes falling one after the other until they hit the final, catastrophic "Migraine Attack" domino.

This is The Domino Effect.

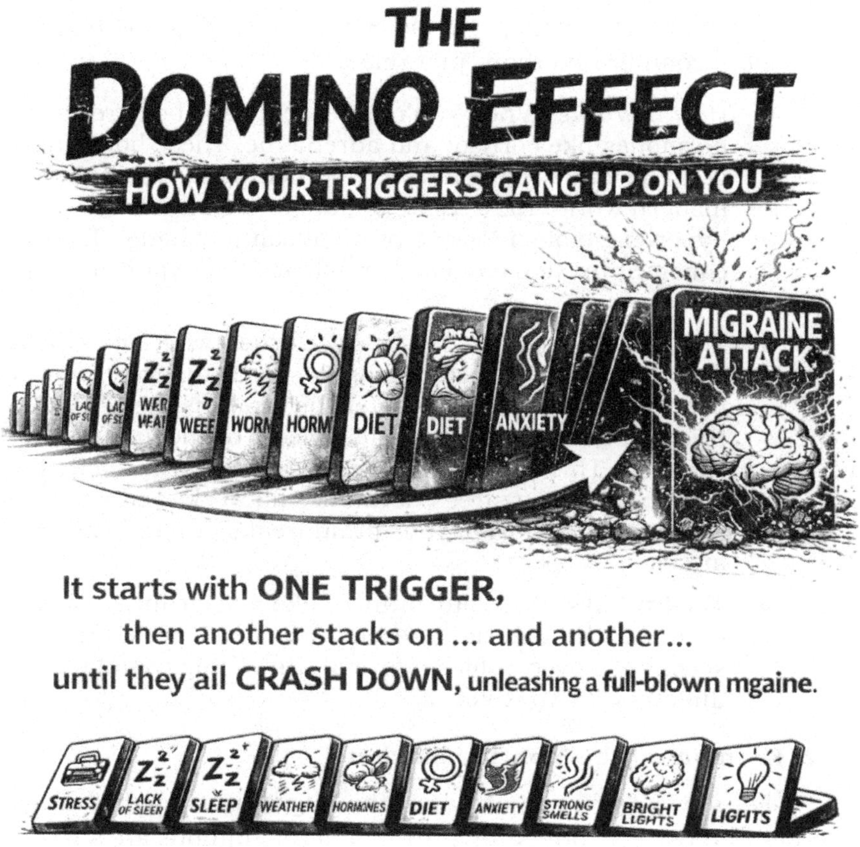
THE
DOMINO EFFECT
HOW YOUR TRIGGERS GANG UP ON YOU
MIGRAINE ATTACK
DIET
DIET
ANXIETY
It starts with ONE TRIGGER,
then another stacks on ... and another...
until they ail CRASH DOWN, unleasling a full-blown mgaine.
STRESS
LACK OF SIEER
SLEEP
WEATHER
HORMONES
DIET
ANXIETY
STRONG SMELLS
BRIGHT LIGHTS
LIGHTS

This image was created with the help of AI.

1. Stress (The Obvious Overlord)

This is the big one, the trigger that everyone---from your doctor to your clueless Aunt Karen---loves to point out. And for once, Aunt Karen isn't entirely wrong. Stress is a massive migraine trigger. But it's more complicated than "just relax."

- How it Works: When you're stressed, your body releases hormones like cortisol and adrenaline. These hormones are great for outrunning a saber-toothed tiger, but in the modern world, they create a state of high alert that your hyper-excitable migraine brain absolutely hates. This constant tension can easily push you over your migraine threshold.
- The "Let-Down" Effect: Here's the cruel twist. The attack doesn't always happen during the stressful event. For many people, the migraine hits after the stress is over---on a Friday afternoon after a hellish week, or the first day of vacation. This is the "let-down headache." Your body has been running on stress hormones all week, and when those levels suddenly drop, your brain freaks out and triggers an attack.
- The Snarky Take: Your brain is like a disgruntled employee. It suffers through the stressful project all week, but the second it's over, it files a formal, throbbing complaint directly with your skull.

2. Hormones (The Monthly Mayhem)

For anyone who menstruates, this trigger is as predictable as the tides and twice as punishing. Hormonal fluctuations are a key driver of migraines, which is a major reason why women are three times more likely to be migraine warriors than men.

- How it Works: The primary culprit is the dramatic drop in estrogen that occurs right before your period. This sudden hormonal shift is believed to lower your migraine threshold, making your brain much more vulnerable to all the other triggers you might encounter. It's like your brain's defensive walls just crumbled, leaving it open to attack. These menstrual migraines are often more severe and harder to treat than migraines at other times of the month.
- Other Hormonal Culprits: It's not just your period. Ovulation, perimenopause, pregnancy, and hormonal birth

control can all mess with your estrogen levels and trigger attacks.

- The Snarky Take: Your hormones are running a protection racket. Pay the estrogen tax or the brain gets it. And the timing is impeccable—because what you really needed alongside cramps and societal expectations was a neurological meltdown on top.

3. Food (The Delicious Deceivers)

Ah, food triggers. The most debated, most personal, and most frustrating category of them all. What triggers one person might be a safe food for another. Finding your specific food triggers is a journey of meticulous detective work.

The Usual Suspects: While personal, some foods are more likely to be villains:

- Aged Cheeses, Cured Meats, and Fermented Foods: These contain high levels of tyramine, an amino acid that can cause blood vessels to constrict and then expand, triggering a vascular headache in some people.

Alcohol: Especially red wine, which contains tyramine, sulfites, and tannins---a triple threat of trigger components.

- **Caffeine:** The ultimate frenemy. For some, a cup of coffee can help stop an attack. For others, too much caffeine is a trigger. And for many, caffeine withdrawal is the real killer.

Artificial Sweeteners: Aspartame is a notorious trigger for some, messing with neurotransmitter levels.

MSG (Monosodium Glutamate): This flavor enhancer can overexcite neurons in the brain, leading to an attack.

- **The Snarky Take:** Food triggers are your body's way of ensuring you can't have nice things. That charcuterie board? A minefield. That glass of Cabernet? A ticking time bomb. Enjoy your plain crackers and water.

4. Environment (The World Is Trying to Hurt You)

Sometimes, it feels like the very atmosphere around you is conspiring to cause an attack. And you're not wrong. Your hyper-sensitive brain is constantly scanning the environment for threats.

How it Works:

- Bright or Flickering Lights: Fluorescent lights, strobing effects, or even bright, glary sunlight can overstimulate your visual cortex, kicking off the CSD wave.
- **Loud Noises:** A loud concert or even just a chronically noisy office can put your auditory system on high alert, contributing to your overall trigger load.
- **Strong Smells (Osmophobia):** Perfumes, cleaning products, gasoline---strong odors can directly activate the trigeminal nerve.
- **Weather Changes:** This is a big one. Many warriors are human barometers. A sudden drop in barometric pressure (which often precedes a storm) can trigger an attack, though the exact mechanism is still being studied.
- **The Snarky Take:** Congratulations, you have a useless superpower. You can predict the weather with your face. The only problem is, the prediction method is debilitating pain.

5. Sleep (The Finicky Foundation)

Sleep is the foundation of a healthy brain. When that foundation is cracked, everything else starts to crumble. Your migraine brain is a total diva about its sleep schedule.

- **How it Works:** Both too little and too much sleep can be potent triggers. Lack of sleep increases stress hormones and inflammation. Oversleeping disrupts your normal circadian rhythm and can throw your brain chemistry out of whack. Consistency is king. Your brain wants you to go to bed and wake up at the same time, every single day. Yes, even on weekends.
- **The Snarky Take:** Your brain demands a perfectly consistent 8-hour sleep schedule with no exceptions. It's like living with a tiny, unreasonable CEO who controls your well-being and has a zero-tolerance policy for hitting the snooze button.

6. Dehydration (The Simplest Saboteur)

This is the trigger that makes you feel the most foolish when it gets you. It's so simple, yet so effective.

- **How it Works:** When you're dehydrated, your blood volume decreases. This can cause your blood vessels to narrow, reducing blood flow to the brain. Your brain, ever the drama queen, interprets this as a major crisis. Even mild dehydration can irritate the meninges (the sensitive lining of the brain), triggering pain.

- **The Snarky Take:** You forgot to drink water, so your brain has decided to punish you with the pain of a thousand suns. Seems like a proportional response.

🕮 Ken's Corner: When Your Body Is the Trigger

Most trigger guides focus on food, sleep, and stress. But for some of us, the trigger hiding in plain sight is physical activity — not exercise in the abstract, but specific movements that load the neck and shoulders. Crawling under a car. Bending over a workbench. Carrying heavy boxes. Overhead work. These aren't on any standard trigger checklist, but they were some of my most reliable migraine triggers for years. If your attacks seem connected to physical loading rather than the usual suspects, track those activities alongside everything else. Note the specific positions and how long you held them. The pattern may point to a structural contributor worth discussing with your doctor — especially if you have any history of neck problems or cervical imaging findings. See Chapters 2 and 7 for more on the cervical-migraine connection.

The "Under-the-Radar" Culprits: The Sneaky Saboteurs

Beyond the Big Six, there's a whole world of subtle, sneaky triggers that might be contributing to your migraine load without you even realizing it. These are the assassins that slip past your defenses because you're not looking for them. Let's unmask a few.

❤ A Note to Your Inner Circle: You Might Be a Trigger Too -- And That's Fixable

This is not an accusation. It's an invitation.

If you live or work closely with someone who has migraines, there's a reasonable chance that some of your normal behaviors -- the things you do every day without thinking -- are landing in their trigger bucket. Strong cologne or perfume. Cooking something pungent when they're already symptomatic. Playing music or TV at a volume that seems totally normal to you. Scheduling demanding social events at the end of their high-stress week. Keeping all the lights blazing in shared spaces.

None of this is your fault. You didn't know. Now you do.

A few small, completely non-sacrificial adjustments can meaningfully reduce how often the bucket overflows. Ask them which environmental factors hit hardest. Ask whether there are specific times of day or week when their threshold tends to run low. Ask what a low-trigger evening looks like, and whether you can occasionally make that happen.

You don't have to become a silent hermit living in the dark. You just have to care enough to ask the questions -- and then actually do the thing they tell you.

That's it. That's the whole ask.

Chapter Four Conclusion: From Victim to Detective

And there you have it. You've walked through the minefield and inspected the dominoes. The world of triggers is complex, personal, and frankly, a bit of a pain in the ass. It can feel overwhelming, like you have to control every single aspect of your life to avoid an attack.

But that's not the goal. Remember, the goal isn't perfection; it's awareness.

This chapter is not a list of things you must now fear and avoid forever. It is a list of suspects. Your job now is not to become a hermit, but to become a detective. Your mission, should you choose to accept it, is to observe, to track, and to find your own personal patterns.

Notice how the dominoes fall in your own life. Is it the night of poor sleep that sets you up for failure, making you vulnerable to the stressful meeting the next day? Is it the hormonal dip that fills your bucket halfway, making that single glass of wine the final, catastrophic trigger?

The actionable advice is this: Stop blaming the last domino that fell. The final trigger that tipped you over the edge is rarely the sole culprit. It was just the final straw. The real power comes from looking back at the entire chain reaction and asking, "Which of these earlier dominoes could I have removed?" Maybe you couldn't avoid the stressful meeting, but you could have prioritized sleep the night before. Maybe you couldn't control the weather, but you could have been extra vigilant about hydration.

This is how you dodge the dominoes. You don't have to dodge all of them. You just have to dodge enough of them to keep your bucket from overflowing.

In the next chapter, we're going to give you the tools to do just that. We're going to build your personal "Migraine Dashboard"---your detective's toolkit for tracking the clues and finally solving the mystery of your own beautiful, complicated, and rebellious brain.

Chapter 5: The Migraine Dashboard

Your Personal Brain-Data HQ

Alright, detective, you've met the villains and you've seen their playbook. You know that migraine attacks aren't random ambushes; they are the result of a carefully orchestrated series of unfortunate events---a cascade of falling dominoes.

So, what now? Now, you stop being the victim of the crime and start being the lead investigator. You trade in your fear for a magnifying glass. To do that, every good detective needs an intelligence-gathering headquarters, a place to pin up clues, track suspects, and connect the red strings of conspiracy.

Welcome to your Migraine Dashboard.

The single most infuriating thing about migraines is how they make you feel powerless, like a hostage to your own brain's whims. The Dashboard is how you take that power back. It's a personalized tracking system designed to turn your vague feelings and frustrating symptoms into cold, hard data. And data, my friend, is ammunition.

Why? Because you can't manage what you don't measure. You can't fight an enemy whose tactics you don't understand. And you certainly can't walk into a doctor's office with a desperate plea of, "My head just hurts a lot," and expect to get a targeted, effective treatment plan. But if you walk in and say, "I've had 12 migraine days in the last 30 days, 80% of which were preceded by less than six hours of sleep and a drop in barometric pressure, and my triptan only works 50% of the time when taken after the pain level hits 6/10," you are no longer a patient. You are a collaborator. You are a data scientist. You are a force to be reckoned with.

This chapter is your step-by-step guide to building that Dashboard. We'll cover the tools, the techniques, and the mindset you need to become the world's foremost expert on the most important subject there is: your own brain.

Choosing Your Weapon: The Detective's Toolkit

Every investigator has their preferred tools. Some like the old-school charm of a notepad and pen; others prefer the high-tech efficiency of a supercomputer. There's no right or wrong answer---only what works for you. Your mission is to choose a weapon you will actually use. Consistency is everything. A half-assed diary is useless. A forgotten app is just taking up space on your phone. Choose your tool, and commit to it like it's the only thing standing between you and the next neurological apocalypse. Because, frankly, it is.

Option A: The Old-School Detective --- The Paper Diary

This is the classic, the analog, the romantic choice. It's you, a pen, and a notebook, documenting the clues of your condition like a hard-boiled detective in a film noir.

The Pros:

- Infinitely Customizable: You are limited only by the laws of paper and ink. You can design your layout, create your own shorthand, and track whatever esoteric symptom you want without waiting for a developer to add it to an app.
- Forces Mindfulness: The physical act of writing something down forces you to pause and be present with your symptoms and circumstances. It can create a deeper connection to the data you're logging.
- Zero Tech Required: No batteries to die, no software updates to run, no data privacy policies to ignore. It's blissfully low-tech. Your diary will never sell your data to advertisers who then try to sell you "migraine-friendly" pillows.
- It's Tangible: You can hold your data in your hands. You can physically flip through the pages and see your journey, which can be incredibly powerful.

The Cons:

- It's a Hassle: Carrying a notebook everywhere is a pain. You're less likely to log an attack in the moment if you have to dig a diary and pen out of your bag, especially when your head is pounding.
- Manual Labor: The analysis is all on you. You have to manually comb through pages of data to spot patterns. This

is difficult on a good day and a near-impossible task when you're wrestling with postdrome brain fog.

It Can Get Lost: Lose the notebook, and you lose your entire case file. There's no cloud backup for your Moleskine.

- The Snarky Take: The paper diary is for the purist, the artisan, the warrior who enjoys the aesthetic of documenting their own suffering. It's for those who want to feel like a 1940s detective solving a case, even if the case is "Why does cheese hate me?" and the detective work is interrupted by frequent bouts of nausea.

Option B: The High-Tech Operative --- Migraine Tracking Apps

This is the modern approach. It's you and your phone, leveraging the power of technology to outsource the tedious parts of detective work. Your smartphone is already your life's command center; why not make it your migraine HQ, too?

The Pros:

- Ultimate Convenience: Your phone is always with you. Logging a migraine takes a few taps, meaning you're far more likely to do it consistently, even in the middle of an attack.
- Automated Intelligence: This is the game-changer. Most apps automatically pull in data like the weather, barometric pressure, and air quality for your location. No need for you to be a human barometer.
- Effortless Analysis: The app is your data scientist sidekick. It crunches the numbers for you and spits out beautiful, easy-to-read reports, charts, and "heat-maps" that show you exactly what your top triggers and most effective treatments are.

Smart Features: Medication reminders, symptom predictions, and community forums are often built right in.

The Cons:

- Screen Time as a Trigger: The irony is not lost on us. If bright screens are a major trigger for you, using an app during an attack might feel like poking the bear. (Though many apps have a "dark mode" for this reason).

- Data Privacy: You are handing over your most sensitive health information to a company. It's crucial to choose reputable apps with clear, transparent privacy policies.
- Option Overload: Some apps can be so feature-rich that they feel overwhelming at first. It can take time to customize them to track only what matters to you.

The Apps to Know:

- Migraine Buddy: This is the undisputed heavyweight champion of migraine apps. It's incredibly comprehensive, allowing you to track every conceivable aspect of your attacks. Its reporting features are top-notch, and it has a massive, active community of fellow warriors, which can be a lifeline on its own.
- Bearable: This app is the holistic choice. It's not just for migraines; it's for tracking your entire health experience. You can log mood, symptoms, energy levels, diet, activities, and more. Its power lies in its ability to show you correlations you might never have spotted otherwise. If you have comorbidities like POTS or Fibromyalgia alongside your migraines, Bearable is brilliant for seeing how all your conditions interact.
- The Snarky Take: An app is for the warrior who believes in working smarter, not harder. Why manually cross-reference your food log with the weather report when you can have a tiny robot in your pocket do it for you, freeing you up to focus on more important tasks, like finding the perfect ice pack-to-forehead angle?

What to Track (and Why It Matters): Your Intelligence Gathering Checklist

Okay, Detective, you've chosen your weapon. Now it's time to decide what information you're actually going to collect. A vague report is a useless report. We need specifics. We need data points so rich and detailed that they tell a story. Here's your official intelligence gathering checklist.

The Core Data (The Non-Negotiables)

This is the absolute baseline. If you track nothing else, track this.

- Date, Start Time, and End Time: This is fundamental. It helps you calculate the frequency and duration of your attacks, which is critical information for your doctor to determine if your condition is episodic or chronic.

- Pain Intensity (1-10 Scale): This needs to be consistent. Establish your own personal scale and stick to it. A "7" for you should mean the same thing every time. When you show your doctor a chart showing your average pain level went from 8 to 5 after starting a new preventive, that is powerful data.
- Location of Pain: Is it unilateral (one side) or bilateral (both sides)? Is it behind the eye? In the temple? Across the whole head? This helps identify which type of migraine or headache disorder you might be dealing with.
- Associated Symptoms: What else happened? Nausea? Vomiting? Aura? Light sensitivity? Sound sensitivity? Dizziness? Brain fog? The complete symptom picture is your fingerprint for this attack.
- Medications Taken: What did you take, at what dose, and at what point in the attack? Did it work? Rate the effectiveness. This data will save you thousands of hours of confusion at doctor's appointments.

The Contextual Data (The Detective Work)

This is where you put on your Sherlock hat and go hunting for the conspiracy.

- Sleep: How many hours did you sleep the night before? What was the quality (a simple 1-5 rating works)? Did you wake up at your usual time?
- Food and Hydration: Log what you ate and drank in the 24 hours before the attack. You don't need to be obsessive, but note anything unusual. This is how you catch the sneaky food triggers.

Stress Level: A simple 1-10 rating for the previous 24 hours. You don't need to write an essay.

- Physical Activity: Did you exercise? Do anything physically demanding? (Remember our friend in Chapter 4 who was crawling under cars.)
- Weather/Environment: Note any obvious changes. Was there a storm? Unusually bright day? New smells or strong fragrances at work?

- Hormonal Notes: For those who menstruate, note the day of your cycle. This data is gold for identifying the hormonal pattern.

The "Connect the Dots" Column

At the end of each entry, leave space for a free-form "my trigger theory" note. After the attack is over, and you're in the postdrome, write down your best guess as to what caused it. Don't censor yourself. Even if you think it was stress combined with the fact that your neighbor mowed his lawn at 7 AM and you ate leftover pizza -- - write it down. Over time, your theories will either be confirmed or refuted by the data, and you'll become a sharper and sharper detective.

Reading Your Intelligence Reports: The Heat-Map

Once you've been tracking for a month or more, it's time to look at the big picture. This is where your app becomes your powerful AI sidekick. These apps take all your manually entered data and turn it into simple, visual reports that do the heavy lifting for you. This is your heat-map, your brain's report card. It tells you, in no uncertain terms, what's working and what is absolutely, unequivocally, not.

Your potential migraine report:

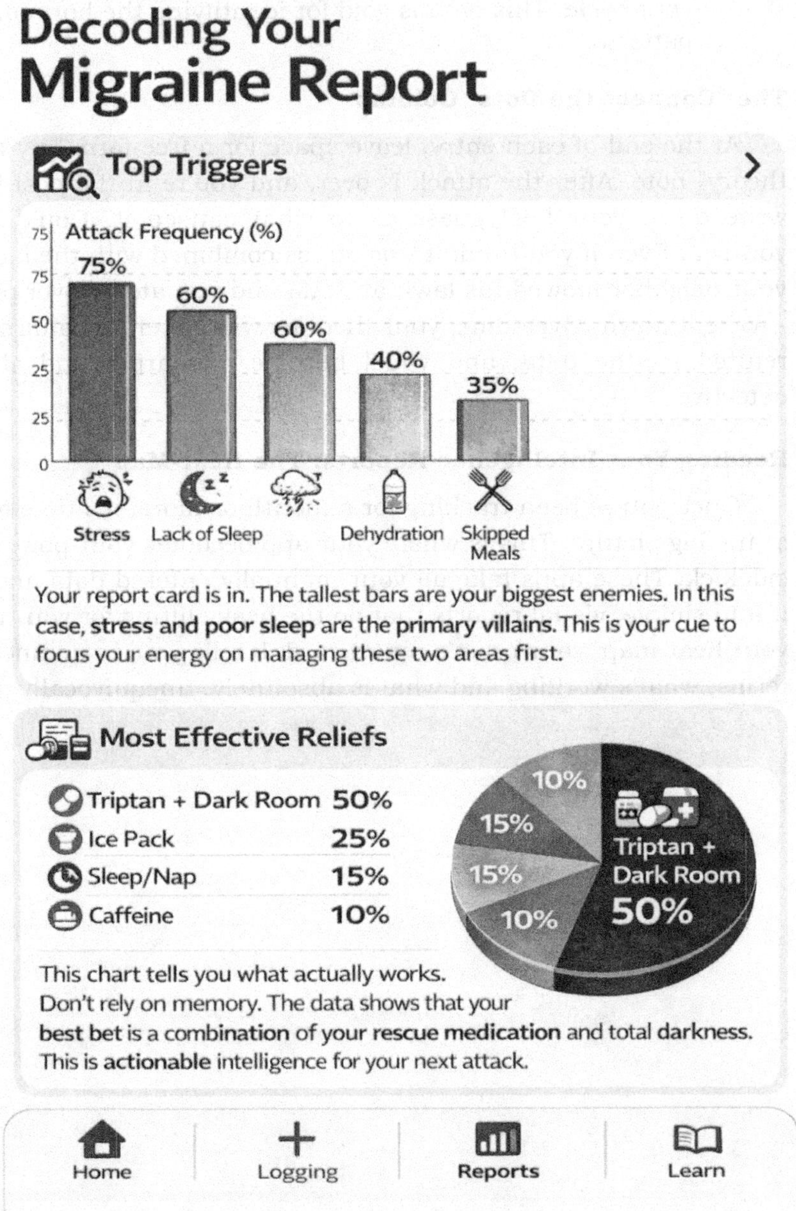

This image was created with the help of AI.

- Confirm Your Suspicions: Did you always have a hunch that rainy days were bad for you? If the "Barometric Pressure" trigger shows up with a high percentage, your hunch is now an evidence-backed fact.
- Discover the Unexpected: You might be surprised by what the data reveals. Maybe you thought chocolate was a trigger, but the data shows it only precedes 5% of your attacks, while "Skipped Lunch" is at 50%. You've been blaming the wrong suspect!
- Track Your Treatment Effectiveness: This is a goldmine for your doctor's appointments. If your report shows that "Triptan A" only provides relief 30% of the time, that's a powerful, objective reason to ask your doctor about trying "Triptan B" or a CGRP-blocker instead.

The heat-map and reports are your cheat sheet. They are the summary of your investigation, a clear and undeniable picture of your brain's patterns. Use them.

The Tools of the Trade: Your Printable Case File

For those who prefer the tangible satisfaction of a paper diary, or for those who want a backup to their app, we've created the ultimate tool. This isn't just a diary; it's a professional-grade case file.

A potential daily migraine log/diary:

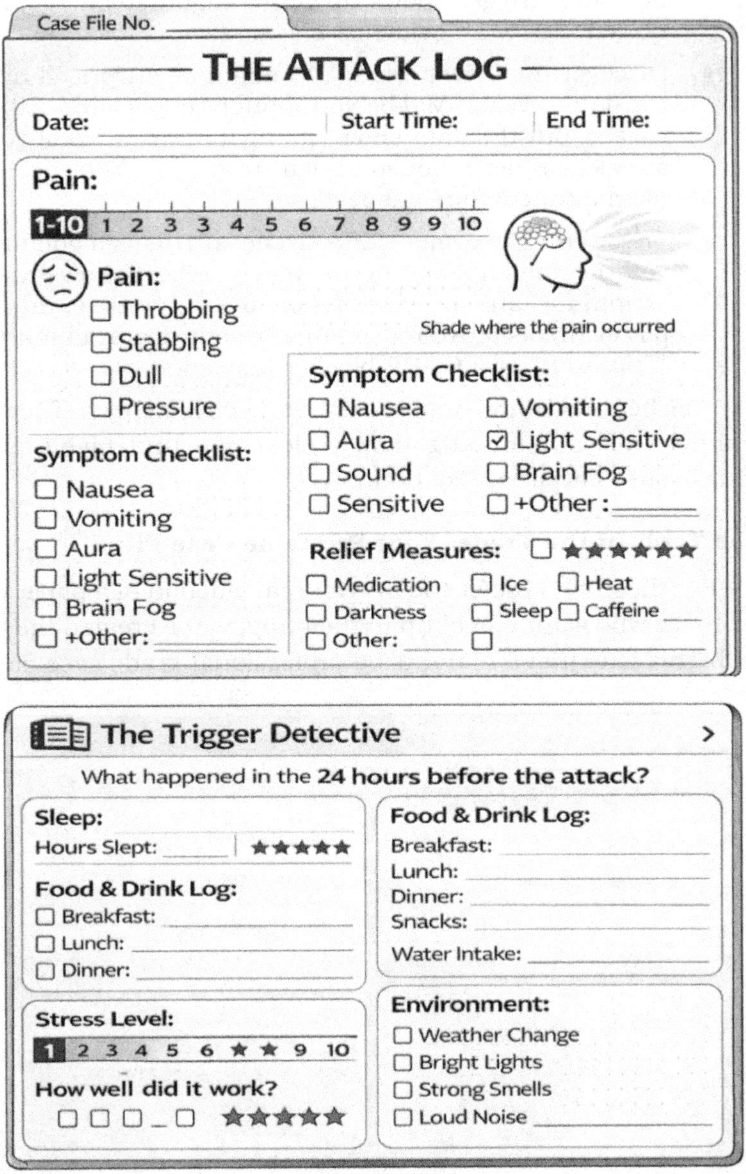

Case File No. ________

THE ATTACK LOG

Date: ________ | Start Time: ____ | End Time: ____

Pain:

1-10 1 2 3 3 4 5 6 7 8 9 9 10

Shade where the pain occurred

Pain:
☐ Throbbing
☐ Stabbing
☐ Dull
☐ Pressure

Symptom Checklist:
☐ Nausea
☐ Vomiting
☐ Aura
☐ Light Sensitive
☐ Brain Fog
☐ +Other: ________

Symptom Checklist:
☐ Nausea ☐ Vomiting
☐ Aura ☑ Light Sensitive
☐ Sound ☐ Brain Fog
☐ Sensitive ☐ +Other: ________

Relief Measures: ☐ ★★★★★★
☐ Medication ☐ Ice ☐ Heat
☐ Darkness ☐ Sleep ☐ Caffeine ____
☐ Other: ____ ☐ ________

The Trigger Detective >

What happened in the **24 hours before the attack?**

Sleep:
Hours Slept: ____ | ★★★★★

Food & Drink Log:
☐ Breakfast: ________
☐ Lunch: ________
☐ Dinner: ________

Food & Drink Log:
Breakfast: ________
Lunch: ________
Dinner: ________
Snacks: ________
Water Intake: ________

Stress Level:
1 2 3 4 5 6 ★ ★ 9 10

How well did it work?
☐ ☐ ☐ _ ☐ ★★★★★

Environment:
☐ Weather Change
☐ Bright Lights
☐ Strong Smells
☐ Loud Noise ________

Image was created with the help of AI.

Your Downloadable Template

Here it is. The key to your new detective agency. Scan this QR code with your phone's camera, and it will take you to a downloadable, beautifully designed, two-page printable PDF of the Ultimate Migraine Diary. It has everything we just talked about, laid out with clean icons, logical columns, and enough space for you to document your descent into madness... I mean, your migraine journey. Print out a stack. Put them in a binder. This is your official case file.

Conclusion: You Are Now the Data-Driven Warrior

Let's be clear. Tracking your migraines is not a cure. It will not magically make the pain disappear. But it ends the guessing game. It replaces helplessness with evidence.

So here is the only question that matters: what did your last three attacks have in common? If you can't answer that yet, open your app or print your diary page tonight. The answer is in the data. Go find it. In the next part of this book, PART III: ACT, we turn that data into a plan you can use.

🕮 Ken's Corner: The Data That Finally Connected the Dots

For nearly five years, I tracked my symptoms the old-fashioned way — in my head. It wasn't until I started documenting everything systematically that the real pattern emerged. The data showed a clear correlation between specific physical activities and my worst attacks. That's what ultimately led me to the structural diagnosis described in Chapter 2. Your data might tell a completely different story. The point is: you won't know until you track it.

Chapter 6: The Acute Attack Playbook

How to Shut It Down FAST

Alright, warrior. Let's get real. The previous chapters were about understanding, anticipating, and becoming a migraine psychic. That's the strategic, long-term work. It's important. It's empowering.

But right now, none of that matters.

Because the Four Horsemen are at your gates. The Ominous Whisper has turned into a roar, the Unwanted Light Show is in full swing, or the first throb of pain has just landed behind your eye with the subtlety of a tactical nuke. The enemy is here. This is not a drill.

Welcome to Part III: ACT. This is where we stop strategizing and start fighting.

This chapter is your emergency manual. Your in-case-of-neurological-fire-break-glass guide. Your Acute Attack Playbook. This is the one chapter I want you to read before you need it, internalize it, and have it ready to deploy at a moment's notice. There is no fluff here. There is only action. Our goal is singular: shut the attack down. Fast.

Forget everything else you've read about long-term management. When the alarms are blaring, you have one job: execute the playbook. Let's go to war.

The "Code Red" Protocol: Your First 15 Minutes

The first 15 minutes of a migraine attack are the most critical battlefield you will ever face. The actions you take in this tiny window can mean the difference between a few hours of manageable misery and a three-day-long neurological hostage crisis.

Your brain is a cascade of chemical reactions. Right now, the first domino has fallen, and a flood of CGRP and other inflammatory villains is just starting to pour out, ready to turn your head into an inflammatory swamp. Our mission is to build a dam and stop that flood before it gets out of control.

You do not have time to "wait and see if it gets worse." You do not have time to be a hero and "power through." When you feel the unmistakable signs of an attack, you initiate the Code Red Protocol immediately. It has three simple, non-negotiable steps: Medicate. Hydrate. Isolate.

Step 1: MEDICATE

This is your first and most powerful counter-attack. The goal of your acute medication is not just to dull the pain; it's to intervene in the biological cascade that causes the pain. Think of it as sending in a special-ops team to neutralize the Chemical Warrior (CGRP) before he can arm all his inflammatory bombs. Timing is everything. Taking your medication early is crucial. Taking it late is like trying to put out a forest fire with a squirt gun.

But what do you take? Your choice of weapon depends on one key question.

Your potential decision tree:

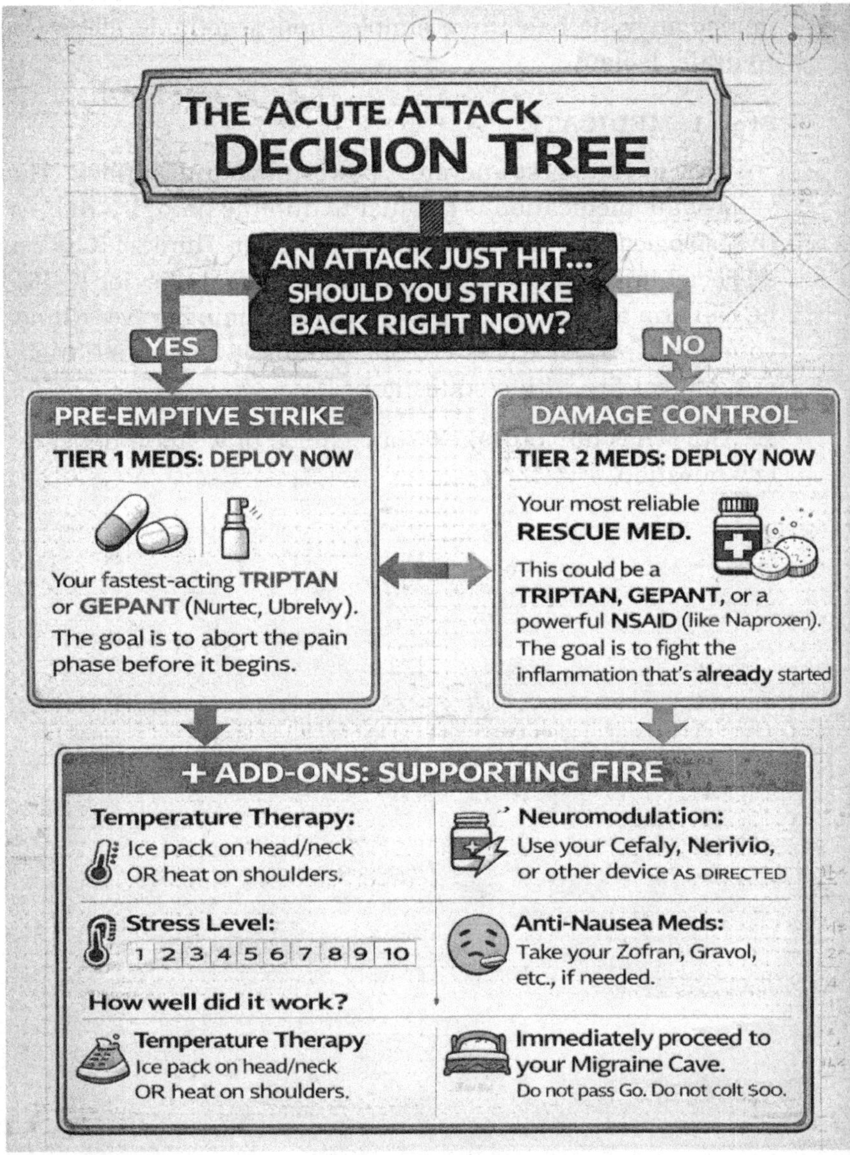

This image was created with the help of AI.

A quick but vital note: This playbook assumes you have worked with a doctor to establish which medications are safe and effective for you. This is not the time to experiment. Use the plan you and your doctor have already created.

Step 2: HYDRATE

The second you've taken your medication, grab some water. But do it strategically. Dehydration thickens your blood and irritates the sensitive tissues around your brain, essentially adding fuel to the inflammatory fire.

However, chugging a giant glass of ice-cold water when you're already feeling nauseous is a rookie mistake that will likely lead to you inspecting the contents of your stomach in the toilet bowl. We're not doing that.

The Right Way to Hydrate:

Sip, don't chug. Take small, gentle sips of room-temperature or cool (not ice-cold) water.

- Add electrolytes. This is a pro-level move. An electrolyte drink (like Pedialyte, Liquid I.V., or even just a pinch of salt and a squeeze of lemon in your water) can help your body absorb the fluid more efficiently and support proper nerve function.
- Ginger is your friend. If nausea is already setting in, try sipping on some weak ginger tea or flat ginger ale. Ginger is a natural anti-emetic.

Your goal is to get about 8-12 ounces of fluid into your system within the first 15-30 minutes. This is a supporting action, but a crucial one.

Step 3: ISOLATE

This is the final step of the Code Red protocol. You have medicated and hydrated. Now, you must retreat from the world. Your brain is in a state of extreme sensory hypersensitivity. Every photon of light and every decibel of sound is a physical assault. You must remove all sensory input immediately.

- Find Your Migraine Cave: You should have a pre-designated space in your home that is your sanctuary. A bedroom, a den, even a walk-in closet in a pinch. It must be a space you can make as dark and as quiet as humanly possible.

- Go Dark: This means turning off all lights, closing all blinds and curtains (blackout curtains are a warrior's best friend), and putting your phone away. The light from a screen is a potent trigger.
- Embrace Silence: Turn off the TV, the music, the fan. Ask your family or roommates to be quiet. If you can't get total silence, use earplugs or noise-canceling headphones.

Medicate. Hydrate. Isolate. This is the trifecta. This is your mantra for the first 15 minutes. Do these three things swiftly and without hesitation, and you have given yourself the best possible chance of shortening the attack and reducing its severity.

Your In-Attack Toolkit: The Tools of the Trade

You are now isolated in your migraine cave, waiting for the medication to work its magic. This is where your non-pharmaceutical toolkit comes into play. These are the tools that provide comfort, offer additional relief, and help you endure the battle ahead.

1. Temperature Therapy: The Great Ice vs. Heat Debate

This is one of the oldest and most effective tricks in the book. But should you use ice or heat? The answer is: it depends on what your brain is screaming for. They work in opposite ways, for different reasons.

The Case for Ice (Fighting the Fire):

- How it Works: Applying cold to your head and neck is a vasoconstrictor---it makes the blood vessels narrow. This directly counteracts the work of the Vascular Mayhem horseman, whose goal is to make those vessels swell and throb. The cold also has a numbing effect on the superficial nerves, which helps dull the pain signals being sent to your brain.

Where to Apply It:

- The Forehead and Temples: Classic placement for a reason. It feels good and targets the branches of the trigeminal nerve.
- The Base of the Skull/Back of the Neck: This is a power move. This area is where your occipital nerves are. Cooling them down can calm irritation and reduce pain signals radiating up your scalp.
- The Carotid Arteries (Sides of your Neck): Cooling the major arteries that send blood to your brain can sometimes help reduce the throbbing.
- The Tools: Gel-based ice packs that conform to your head are fantastic. A "headache hat" or wrap that you can wear is even better, as it provides gentle compression and frees up your hands. In a pinch? A bag of frozen peas is a time-honored cliché for a reason. It works.

The Case for Heat (Relaxing the Tension):

- How it Works: While cold constricts, heat does the opposite: it relaxes. Applying heat to tight muscles, particularly in your neck and shoulders, increases blood flow and helps them release tension. Many migraines are accompanied or exacerbated by severe muscle tension in the cervical region. Releasing these muscles can alleviate a major secondary source of pain.

Where to Apply It:

- Across the Shoulders and Upper Back: Drape a heating pad here to melt away the tension that builds up when you're hunched over in pain.

On the Back of the Neck: A warm compress can soothe tight suboccipital muscles.

- Never directly on your throbbing temple. You want to constrict the blood vessels in your head, not dilate them further. Heat is for the supporting muscles, not the main event.
- The Pro-Gamer Move: The Combo Attack: Some warriors swear by using both. An ice pack on the head to fight the vascular pain, and a heating pad on the shoulders to release the muscle tension. It's the ultimate temperature-based pincer movement. Listen to your body. It will tell you what it needs.

2. Darkness & Silence: The Sensory Deprivation Strategy

Your brain on migraine is like a microphone with the gain turned all the way up. It's picking up everything, and it's all coming through as painful, distorted feedback. This isn't just you being "sensitive"; it's a physiological reality of the attack. Your thalamus, the brain's central relay station for sensory information, is going haywire. It's lost its ability to filter incoming signals, so every photon of light and every sound wave hits your brain with the force of a physical blow.

The only logical response is to cut off the supply. This is not about comfort; it's about removing the fuel that is actively making the attack worse.

The Power of True Darkness: We're not talking "dimly lit." We are talking "cave-on-a-moonless-night" dark.

- Blackout Curtains: These are not a luxury; they are a medical necessity for a migraine warrior. Invest in good ones that block every sliver of light.
- The Eye Mask: For when you can't control the room's lighting (or for daytime attacks), a good eye mask is your best friend. Pro-tip: get a contoured one that doesn't put pressure directly on your eyeballs. It feels less claustrophobic and does a better job of blocking out peripheral light. Some are even weighted or can be chilled in the freezer for a double-whammy of relief.

The Sanctuary of Silence:

- Earplugs: The simplest and most effective tool for blocking out the world. Keep them everywhere: your bedside table, your car, your work bag.
- Noise-Canceling Headphones: This is the next level. True active noise cancellation doesn't just block sound; it creates an envelope of pure, blissful silence. It can be a game-changer for surviving in a house with other living beings (like children or partners who breathe too loudly).
- The White Noise Counter-Attack: For some people, absolute silence can be unnerving and actually make tinnitus (ringing in the ears), a common migraine symptom, more noticeable. In this case, a white noise machine or an app playing gentle, non-looping sounds (like rain or a fan) can mask the jarring, unpredictable noises of the outside world,

creating a predictable and soothing soundscape for your brain to latch onto.

3. Neuromodulation Widgets: Your Sci-Fi Arsenal

Welcome to the future of migraine treatment. If medications are your chemical warfare, neuromodulation devices are your electronic warfare. These gadgets use gentle electrical or magnetic pulses to interact with your nerves and interrupt the pain signals. They are non-invasive, drug-free, and for some, incredibly effective.

Cefaly (The Electric Headband):

- What it is: A device you wear like a futuristic headband. It has an electrode that sticks to your forehead, directly over the primary branches of the trigeminal nerve.
- How it Works (The Acute Setting): When you trigger the "attack" mode, the device sends a high-frequency electrical stimulation to the trigeminal nerve. This stimulation essentially "scrambles" the pain signals. It's like creating static on the phone line between your face and your brain, so the messages of agony can't get through as clearly. It can dull the pain and make the attack more tolerable.
- The Snarky Take: Yes, it looks a bit like you're a lost member of the Borg from Star Trek. But if it means less pain, who cares? You can call yourself Locutus of Migraine. Resistance is, in fact, futile.

Nerivio (The Smart Armband):

- What it is: A device that looks like a modern armband, controlled by an app on your smartphone. You wear it on your upper arm.
- How it Works (This is the cool part): This device uses a fascinating process called Conditioned Pain Modulation (CPM). It delivers gentle electrical pulses to the nerves in your arm. Your brain senses this stimulation and, in response, activates its own built-in, descending pain-inhibition system. Essentially, by creating a non-painful distraction on your arm, you're tricking your brain into turning down the volume of the much more severe pain in your head. It's like telling your brain, "Hey, never mind that five-alarm fire in the skull, we've got this little thing on the arm to deal with." It's a brilliant biological hack.

- The Snarky Take: You're basically using a remote control on your own nervous system to change the channel from "Head Exploding" to "Slightly Tingling Arm." It's the ultimate life hack, and you don't even have to enter a cheat code.

If you have known cervical disease and your attacks are reliably associated with neck-loading activities, the acute playbook above still applies — but your long-term strategy may also need to address the structural source. We cover cervical-specific preventive treatments, including diagnostic injections and physical therapy, in Chapter 7.

The Art of Bailing: A Warrior's Guide to Canceling Plans Without Guilt

This might be the most important skill you learn in this entire book. As a migraine warrior, you will have to cancel plans. You will miss birthday parties. You will bail on date nights. You will ghost work happy hours. This is an unavoidable fact of our existence.

The guilt that comes with this is immense. You feel unreliable, flaky, and like a burden. It's time to surgically remove that guilt from your brain, because it is a useless emotion that serves only to make a bad situation worse.

Canceling is not a personal failure. It is a strategic act of medical self-preservation. You are not "bailing." You are deploying a critical part of your treatment plan. You are choosing your health over a social or professional obligation, and that is not just okay---it is necessary and admirable.

To do it effectively, you need scripts. Memorize them. Practice them. Use them without apology.

The Script for Friends (Casual & Direct):

"Hey, so my brain has decided to betray me today and a nasty migraine is starting. I'm so sorry, but I have to bail on [tonight's awesome plan]. I need to go into my dark cave now before it gets worse. I'm super bummed to miss it. Let's please reschedule for next week?"

- Why it works: It's honest, direct, expresses regret, and immediately proposes a solution (rescheduling), showing you still value the friendship.

The Script for Work (Professional & Boundary-Setting):

"Hi [Boss/Colleague], just wanted to let you know that I have a migraine starting. I need to take my acute medication and go offline for a bit to manage it effectively. I will address [urgent task] as soon as I am able, and I will check back in around [timeframe, e.g., two hours, or tomorrow morning]."

- Why it works: It's professional. It frames the migraine as a medical event you are actively "managing." It sets a clear boundary ("I need to go offline") and provides a reasonable timeframe for your return, which eases your manager's anxiety. You don't need to give details or sound overly apologetic.

The Script for a Partner/Family (Loving & Instructional):

"Hey, my love. It's happening. The Code Red has been initiated. I need to retreat to the bedroom now. Could you please do me a huge favor and [specific, actionable request, e.g., 'make sure the kids keep the volume down' or 'grab my ice pack from the freezer']? Thank you so much. I love you."

- Why it works: It's a clear signal, it tells them exactly how they can help (which makes them feel useful, not helpless), and it ends with affection, reinforcing that your retreat is about your head, not about them.

Dismantle the guilt. Canceling is not a moral failing. It's medicine.

ACTION BOX: When to Go to the ER --- The "Code Black" Checklist

99% of your migraines, however brutal, are not life-threatening. But that other 1% is why this box exists. If you experience ANY of the following, stop everything and go to the emergency room or call for emergency medical help immediately. This is not the time to be a tough guy.

Use the S.N.O.O.P. mnemonic to remember the red flags:

- S - Systemic Symptoms: Your headache is accompanied by a fever, chills, unexplained weight loss, or a stiff neck you can't explain.
- N - Neurologic Signs: You have neurological symptoms you've never had with a migraine before. This includes confusion, seizure, double vision, loss of consciousness, or weakness/numbness that is severe or doesn't go away.

- O - Onset: The headache comes on suddenly and explosively, like being struck by lightning. This is often called a "thunderclap headache" and is a major red flag for a brain bleed. It reaches maximum intensity in under a minute.
- O - Older Age: You are over 50 and this is the first time you have ever had a headache this severe, or it is a brand new type of headache for you.
- P - Pattern Change: This headache is fundamentally different from your usual migraine attacks. The location is new, the intensity is unprecedented, it's getting progressively worse over days, or it's not responding to any treatments that usually work.

The bottom line: Trust your gut. If something feels dangerously wrong and different from your typical migraine, seek immediate medical care. It's always better to be safe than sorry.

Conclusion: Your Battle Plan Is Ready

You've made it through the playbook. You now have a clear, concise, and powerful protocol for the moment the battle begins. Your new mantra: Medicate. Hydrate. Isolate. You have your toolkit ready, from the low-tech power of an ice pack to the sci-fi wizardry of neuromodulation. You have your scripts to navigate the social fallout with grace and self-respect. And most importantly, you know the difference between a Code Red and a Code Black.

This is control. This is power. It's not the power to prevent every attack, but it is the power to fight back intelligently and effectively when one does strike. You have the plan. You have the tools. And you know exactly what to do when the alarms start blaring.

So, here's your final piece of actionable advice for this chapter. Do it right now. Don't wait. Go build your Code Red Kit. Get a small bag and physically put your tools in it. Your go-to rescue medication. A bottle of water and an electrolyte packet. A comfortable eye mask. A good pair of earplugs. This is your migraine go-bag, your emergency kit. Put one in your car, one at your desk, and one by your bed. Be prepared.

You now have the plan for fighting the fires. In the next chapter, we're going to learn how to fireproof the building. Prevention starts now.

Chapter 7: The Preventive Arsenal

Building Your Defenses

The last chapter was your emergency guide—what to do when the Four Horsemen are already ransacking your skull. That was firefighting.

This chapter is about fireproofing.

Welcome to the long game. If the Acute Attack Playbook is your shield and sword, this chapter is where we build the fortress—a defense so formidable that the enemy often decides it's not even worth attacking.

The goal of prevention isn't necessarily to achieve a mythical state of being "migraine-free" forever (though we can dream). The goal is to reduce the frequency, severity, and duration of your attacks. It's to turn a 15-day-a-month war zone into a handful of manageable skirmishes. It's about taking back your calendar and your life from the clutches of chronic pain.

The world of preventive migraine treatment is vast, ranging from simple lifestyle tweaks to high-tech biologic drugs. It can be overwhelming. To make sense of it all, we're going to organize your arsenal into a "Ladder of Therapies." You start with the foundational steps at the bottom, and only climb higher with the guidance of your doctor if needed. Each rung on the ladder represents a step up in intensity and intervention.

Let's start building your fortress.

Tier 1: Lifestyle Rhythms (The Non-Negotiable Foundation)

(Evidence Strength: ★★★★★)

Before we even whisper the word "medication," we have to talk about the foundation upon which all other treatments are built. If you ignore this tier, you are trying to build a castle on a swamp. It doesn't matter how advanced your weapons are if your fortress walls are sinking into the mud. These are the non-negotiables. They are boring, they are not sexy, and they are the most powerful preventive tools you have.

Your migraine brain, as we've established, is a hypersensitive diva. It doesn't like surprises. It craves consistency. It thrives on rhythm and routine. The goal of this tier is to give your brain the predictable, stable environment it needs to stay calm.

- Sleep-Wake Locking: Your brain has a tiny clock in it called the suprachiasmatic nucleus, and it takes its job very seriously. When you mess with your sleep schedule, you throw that clock into a state of jet-lagged chaos. The most powerful thing you can do for your migraine brain is to go to bed and wake up at the same time every single day. Yes, that includes weekends. Yes, it's deeply unfair. Sleeping in until 10 AM on a Saturday might feel like a luxurious reward, but to your brain, it's a shocking disruption that can easily trigger a weekend-ruining attack.
- The Snarky Take: Treat your brain like the world's most demanding toddler. It needs a strict, non-negotiable bedtime. It doesn't care that you want to stay up late to watch one more episode. It will make you pay for it tomorrow with a screaming, head-pounding tantrum.
- Stress Management: Telling a migraine warrior to "just relax" is grounds for justifiable homicide. We're not talking about eliminating stress---that's impossible. We're talking about building your stress resilience. It's about managing your reaction to stress. When you're stressed, your body pumps out cortisol, a hormone that puts your nervous system on high alert---exactly the state a migraine brain hates. Practices like mindfulness, meditation (apps like Headspace or Calm are great), gentle yoga, or even just 10 minutes of deep breathing a day can help regulate your nervous system. They teach your brain that not every stressful email is a saber-toothed tiger that requires a full-scale neurological meltdown.
- The Snarky Take: Think of it as sending your brain to a spa. It doesn't want to go at first. It thinks it's too busy. But after a few minutes of quiet and breathing, it realizes it's not actually being chased by a predator and decides maybe it won't set your head on fire today.
- Hydration: This is so basic it feels insulting, but it is fundamental. We discussed this in the trigger chapter, but from a preventive standpoint, consistent hydration is key.

Dehydration lowers your blood volume and can irritate the sensitive meninges around your brain. Don't wait until you're thirsty. Keep a water bottle with you at all times and sip consistently throughout the day.

- The Snarky Take: Your brain is approximately 75% water. When that level drops, it doesn't send you a polite memo. It sends you a throbbing, pulsating invoice for your negligence, with pain as the late fee.

Tier 2: Supplements & Nutrition (The Over-the-Counter Allies)

(Evidence Strength: ★★★☆☆)

Once your lifestyle foundation is solid, you might consider adding some reinforcements. This tier involves over-the-counter supplements that have shown real promise in clinical studies for migraine prevention. They are generally safer and have fewer side effects than prescription medications, making them an excellent second line of defense.

IMPORTANT CAVEAT: "Natural" does not automatically mean "safe." Always, and I mean always, talk to your doctor before starting any new supplement. They can interfere with other medications or be inappropriate for certain health conditions.

Now, let's meet the support crew.

Magnesium (The "Chill-Out" Mineral):

- How it Works: Magnesium is essential for proper nerve and muscle function. It plays a key role in calming down our old friend, the hyper-excitable brain. It helps block pain-transmitting chemicals and can prevent the CSD wave from starting. Many migraine warriors are found to be deficient in this crucial mineral.
- The Evidence: Multiple studies have shown that a daily magnesium supplement can reduce the frequency and severity of migraine attacks, especially for those with menstrual migraine or migraine with aura.
- Dosage & Form: Doctors typically recommend 400-600 mg per day. Look for forms that are easily absorbed, like magnesium glycinate or magnesium citrate. The cheap stuff, magnesium oxide, will mostly just give you diarrhea, which is not the therapeutic effect we're going for.

- The Snarky Take: Think of magnesium as a bouncer for your brain's nightclub. It stands at the door and tells your over-excited neurons, "Sorry, you're not getting in tonight. Go home and chill out."

Riboflavin (Vitamin B2) (The "Cellular Fuel"):

- How it Works: There's a theory that migraines are, in part, an "energy crisis" in the brain. The mitochondria---the tiny power plants inside your brain cells---might not be working efficiently. Riboflavin is a key component in mitochondrial energy production. The idea is that by giving your brain cells more B2, you're helping them produce energy more effectively, making them more resilient to triggers.
- The Evidence: Clinical trials have shown that a high dose of Riboflavin can be an effective preventive for some people, reducing attack frequency by up to 50%. It's considered safe and well-tolerated.
- Dosage: This requires a high dose to be effective: 400 mg per day. This is way more than you can get from food, so supplementation is necessary. Be warned: it will turn your pee a shocking, neon-highlighter yellow. This is normal and harmless, but it's good to know before you think your body is having a radioactive event.
- The Snarky Take: Taking high-dose B2 is like upgrading the power grid for your brain. Also, the neon pee is a fun party trick and a constant reminder that you are actively fighting your migraines.

Coenzyme Q10 (CoQ10) (The "Mitochondrial Sidekick"):

- How it Works: Similar to B2, CoQ10 is another crucial compound for mitochondrial health and energy production. It also acts as a powerful antioxidant, helping to protect brain cells from inflammatory damage.
- The Evidence: The evidence is less robust than for Magnesium or B2, but several studies have shown it can be beneficial, particularly in children and adolescents, and is often recommended as part of a "migraine cocktail" of supplements.

Dosage: A typical dose is 100-300 mg per day.

- The Snarky Take: If B2 is the main power station, CoQ10 is the skilled engineer making sure everything runs smoothly and efficiently.

A Word on the Herbs: Feverfew & Butterbur:

- Feverfew: A plant that has been used for centuries to treat headaches. It's thought to reduce inflammation. The evidence is mixed, and its effectiveness can vary wildly depending on the preparation and the patient.
- Butterbur: This plant has some of the strongest evidence among herbal remedies for reducing migraine frequency. It's believed to act as an anti-inflammatory and a natural beta-blocker. Read the warning below!
- THE BIG, SCARY WARNING: Standard preparations of butterbur can contain chemicals called pyrrolizidine alkaloids (PAs), which are toxic to the liver. If you ever consider trying butterbur, you must use a brand that is certified PA-free. This is non-negotiable. Do not forage for this in your backyard.
- The Snarky Take: Herbs can be helpful, but they are still drugs. Treat them with respect. Especially the one with the potential to poison your liver. Stick with the PA-free stuff, or just stick with the magnesium. It's less dramatic.

Tier 3: The Classics (The Prescription Heavy Artillery)

(Evidence Strength: ★★★★☆)

Alright, you've solidified your foundation with lifestyle changes and maybe added some supplemental support. But for many of us, that's not enough to keep the Four Horsemen at bay. Sometimes, you need to call in the heavy artillery.

This tier consists of the "classic" prescription medications. These are the time-tested, evidence-backed workhorses that have been used for migraine prevention for decades. Here's the funny thing about most of them: they weren't originally designed for migraine. They are borrowed drugs, repurposed from other medical fields after doctors noticed a happy side effect: they made their patients' migraines better. Think of these as the multi-tool of pharmaceuticals---designed for one job, but surprisingly good at another.

1. Beta-Blockers (e.g., Propranolol, Metoprolol)

- What They Really Are: These drugs were developed to treat high blood pressure and performance anxiety. They work by blocking the effects of adrenaline, slowing your heart rate, and making you feel less like you're about to have a panic attack during a public speaking gig.

- How They Help Migraine: That same calming effect on your cardiovascular system seems to help our cause. By stabilizing blood vessels and reducing the body's overall "fight-or-flight" response, beta-blockers can make your brain less reactive to triggers. They essentially tell your hyper-excitable nervous system to take a deep breath and chill out for a second. They are one of the most common first-line prescription defenses for a reason---they work, and they're generally well-tolerated.
- The Snarky Take: Your doctor is prescribing you a drug designed to stop a rock star from having a heart attack from stage fright. Turns out, your brain on the verge of a migraine acts a lot like a nervous rock star. It's a happy little accident of pharmacology.

2. Antidepressants (e.g., Amitriptyline, Venlafaxine)

- What They Really Are: Let's clear the air on this immediately. When your doctor suggests an antidepressant for your migraines, they are not implying your pain is "all in your head" or that you're "just depressed." This is a common and frustrating misconception. While these drugs do treat depression, they are being used here for a completely different, biological reason.
- How They Help Migraine: These specific classes of antidepressants (tricyclics like amitriptyline and SNRIs like venlafaxine) work by increasing the levels of neurotransmitters like serotonin and norepinephrine in your brain. These chemical messengers don't just regulate mood; they are critical players in regulating your body's pain signaling pathways. By tweaking the levels of these chemicals, you can effectively turn down the volume on pain signals and make the nerves in your brain less likely to overreact.
- The Snarky Take: You're using a mood drug to tell your trigeminal nerve to stop being so damn extra. It's a form of chemical negotiation, convincing your overactive pain pathways that not everything is a catastrophe that requires a full-scale meltdown.

3. Anti-Seizure Medications (e.g., Topiramate, Valproate)

- What They Really Are: As the name suggests, these drugs were developed to prevent seizures in people with epilepsy by calming excessive electrical activity in the brain.
- How They Help Migraine: This one is beautifully direct. Remember our first horseman, The Spark (Neuronal Hyper-excitability)? These drugs ride directly into battle against him. They work by raising your brain's seizure threshold, which in our case means raising the migraine threshold. They make your neurons less twitchy and less likely to fire off the wave of Cortical Spreading Depression that starts the whole mess.
- The Brutal Honesty Section (Side Effects): These medications can be incredibly effective, but they often come with a price. Topiramate, in particular, is infamous for its cognitive side effects, earning it the loving nicknames "Dopamax" or "Stupamax." Users often report significant brain fog, word-finding difficulties (that feeling of a word being on the tip of your tongue, but for every word), and tingling in their hands and feet. For some, the relief from migraine is worth the trade-off. For others, it's not. This is a serious conversation to have with your doctor and your loved ones.
- The Snarky Take: This drug is a bargain with the devil. It might quiet the electrical storm in your head, but it could also make you forget your own zip code. Choose your poison wisely.

☐ From the Clinic: The Two-Birds-One-Stone Approach

*Contributed by **Elliott James, APRN, MSN, CMRD** — Advanced Practice Registered Nurse, Neurology*

Before we climb to the next tier, my own NP, Elliott James, wanted to share something with you that I think is genuinely valuable — and that most patients never hear about in the fifteen minutes they get with their provider.

The CGRP-blocking medications we're about to cover in Tier 4 changed the game for many migraine sufferers worldwide, and they've become the go-to treatment for those significantly affected. But here's what Elliott wants you to know: the classic medications we just covered above? They're not just migraine drugs. In fact, most of them weren't even designed for migraines in the first place. They were invented for other purposes — seizures, depression, high blood pressure — and prescribers realized along the way that they were also helping patients' migraines. So they started using them for that too.

And that's where it gets interesting. Because if you have migraines plus another condition that one of these drugs already treats, a smart provider can kill two birds with one stone — or sometimes even three. Got migraines and depression? Venlafaxine treats both. Migraines and seizures? Topiramate has you covered. Migraines, anxiety, and high blood pressure? Say hello to propranolol.

But we're still not done. Because these drugs also have that usually-dreaded, all-scary word: side effects. Here's the thing, though — sometimes side effects can actually work in your favor. Amitriptyline almost always causes sleepiness, so it's given at bedtime and is a great choice for migraineurs who also have trouble sleeping. Topiramate may curb appetite and is sometimes associated with weight loss — a side effect that should be monitored carefully, and which excludes some patients from being good candidates, but which in some cases can be beneficial (there is data that weight loss can improve migraine management as well).

Here's Elliott's quick-reference guide to the classic migraine medications and their **bonus benefits:**

Topiramate: Migraines, seizures, essential tremor, weight loss.

Amitriptyline and Nortriptyline: Migraines, nerve pain, insomnia, depression, anxiety, some specific GI issues (talk to a GI specialist about that one).

Propranolol: Migraines, high blood pressure, high heart rate and abnormal heart rhythm, anxiety, essential tremor.

Carbamazepine and Oxcarbazepine: Migraines, seizures, other nerve pains (especially trigeminal neuralgia).

Venlafaxine and Duloxetine: Migraines, other nerve pains, depression, anxiety.

Lamotrigine: Migraines, seizures, mood disorders (including depression, anxiety, and bipolar disorder), and it is an excellent choice for ocular migraine without headache (migraine-related vision symptoms).

Gabapentin: Seizures, migraines, almost any kind of nerve pain, essential tremor, restless leg syndrome — this one is the Swiss Army knife of neurology.

A critical note from Elliott: Just because a drug looks like a great fit based on the list above doesn't mean it is. These drugs all have risks, and it's important to know the specifics. For instance, propranolol is likely a bad idea if you have asthma. Amitriptyline is a poor choice if you have a history of certain heart rhythm abnormalities, or if you're on other sedating medications. Topiramate can interact poorly with birth control medications, and is definitely a bad idea if you have a history of kidney stones. The goal is to find a medication that works great for you — but it's most important that, first and foremost, you stay safe with your meds.

The Snarky Take: Think of it this way — you walked into the pharmacy thinking you were picking up one prescription for one problem. Turns out, your provider just wrote you a multi-tool. It's like buying a Swiss Army knife when you only needed a bottle opener — except this one also fixes your sleep, calms your nerves, and tells your trigeminal nerve to sit down and shut up. These intricacies are not usually going to be discussed in great depth during a fifteen-minute office visit, so bring this list to your next appointment and have the conversation with your provider. You might find a single medication that covers a lot more ground than you thought possible.

Tier 4: The New Guard (The Sci-Fi Weapons)

(Evidence Strength: ★★★★★)

If the classic meds are the heavy artillery, this tier is the special forces. These are the new-school, high-tech, targeted therapies that have completely revolutionized migraine prevention in the last decade. They weren't "borrowed" from other fields; they were designed from the ground up with one mission and one mission only: to seek and destroy the specific mechanisms of migraine.

1. CGRP Monoclonal Antibodies (e.g., Aimovig, Ajovy, Emgality)

- What They Are: These are the rock stars of modern migraine treatment. They are laboratory-produced antibodies---highly specific proteins---delivered via an auto-injector pen you use at home, usually once a month or once every three months.
- How They Help Migraine: This is where our intel on the Four Horsemen pays off. Remember the Chemical Warrior, CGRP? The protein that acts as the primary fuel for migraine pain and inflammation? These drugs are literal CGRP assassins. They are engineered to do one of two things: either they act like a sponge and sop up all the excess CGRP floating around your system, or they act as a blocker, sitting on the CGRP receptors so the CGRP can't dock and deliver its message of pain. They stop the chemical siege before it can even begin.
- The Snarky Take: For decades, we carpet-bombed the brain with borrowed drugs, hoping for some collateral benefit. This is the first time in history we've had a laser-guided smart bomb aimed squarely at the head of the bad guy. It's a beautiful thing.

2. Gepants for Prevention (e.g., Qulipta, Nurtec ODT)

- What They Are: Gepants are another class of CGRP-fighters, but they are "small molecule" drugs that come in a pill form. While some gepants are used for acute attacks (as seen in Chapter 6), some are now approved for prevention, taken as a daily or every-other-day pill.
- How They Help Migraine: They do the same job as the monoclonal antibodies---block CGRP from causing chaos---but they do it in a different way. Because they are small molecules, they are cleared from your system much faster. This gives you and your doctor more flexibility. It's a great option for people who are needle-shy or who want a CGRP-blocker they can stop and start more easily.
- The Snarky Take: If the antibody injections are the long-range sniper rifle, gepants are the trusty, everyday sidearm. Different tool, same target.

3. Botox (for Chronic Migraine Only)

- What It Is: Yes, this is the very same botulinum toxin used to smooth wrinkles. But here, it's not being used for cosmetic reasons. It is a powerful, FDA-approved preventive treatment specifically and only for people with chronic migraine (meaning you have 15 or more headache days per month). If you have episodic migraine, this is not the droid you're looking for.

- How It Helps Migraine: It's not about "freezing" your muscles so you can't frown. The Botox is injected in a specific 31-shot pattern around the head and neck. It works by getting into the nerve endings and blocking the release of pain-transmitting chemicals, including our old pal CGRP. It essentially deadens the pain signals at the source, preventing them from ever reaching the brain. The procedure is repeated every 12 weeks.
- The Snarky Take: You're using a neurotoxin to paralyze the pain signals from your own nerves. It's the neurological equivalent of cutting the phone lines before the prank caller can even dial. And as a bonus, you'll have a beautifully smooth, expressionless forehead. It's a win-win, really.

When the Neck Is the Trigger: Targeting the Source

Not every migraine begins purely in the brain. For a surprising number of people, the spark that lights the migraine fuse actually starts lower down the chain, in the neck.

The upper cervical spine is an incredibly busy piece of biological infrastructure. The joints, muscles, and nerves in the C1 through C3 region sit directly upstream of one of the most important migraine control centers in the body: the **trigeminocervical complex**. Think of this structure as a neurological switchboard where signals from the neck and signals from the migraine pathways converge and get sorted.

When the neck is calm, the system works normally. When the neck is irritated, inflamed, or mechanically stressed, that switchboard can start sending the wrong signals.

Years of poor posture, cervical spine degeneration, tight muscles, whiplash injuries, or compressed nerves can irritate the **occipital nerve system**, which runs from the top of your spinal cord up into the scalp. When those nerves get angry, the pain signals they send can travel straight into the trigeminocervical complex and start amplifying the migraine circuitry.

Translation: your neck can light the fuse. And if that fuse burns long enough, the migraine system eventually detonates. This is why so many migraine sufferers report the same strange pattern: the attack seems to begin with neck stiffness, soreness at the base of the skull, or tight shoulders before the full neurological storm arrives.

In those cases, treating the **neck inflammation or nerve irritation directly** can sometimes reduce the intensity of attacks or prevent them from escalating into a full migraine cascade.

There are several tools doctors use when the neck appears to be part of the problem.

Diclofenac Sodium Topical Gel: The Local Anti-Inflammatory Strike

One of the simplest and most targeted treatments for neck-driven headache pain is **topical diclofenac sodium gel**.

Diclofenac is a non-steroidal anti-inflammatory drug (NSAID), but unlike the pills you swallow, this version is delivered directly through the skin to the tissues underneath.

Instead of sending medication throughout your entire body, the drug concentrates in the muscles and joints where the inflammation is actually happening.

That makes it particularly useful for conditions involving the upper cervical spine and surrounding musculature, including irritated neck muscles, mild cervical arthritis, localized nerve irritation, or the chronic muscle tension that develops from years of "tech-neck" posture.

Applied to the base of the skull, the upper neck, or the shoulder muscles, diclofenac gel can help quiet the inflammatory signals that aggravate the occipital nerves. By calming that local inflammation, it sometimes reduces the background irritation that feeds into the migraine system.

Another advantage is that topical NSAIDs generally produce far fewer systemic side effects than oral ones. Because the medication stays mostly local, the stomach irritation and gastrointestinal risks associated with long-term NSAID use are significantly reduced.

Think of it as putting the fire extinguisher directly on the spark instead of spraying the entire building.

Cannabis-Based Topical Creams: The Muscle Relaxation Strategy

Another option that some patients find helpful for neck-driven headache pain is the use of **topical cannabis-based creams**, particularly those containing CBD, THC, or a combination of both.

Unlike oral cannabis products, topical preparations do not significantly enter the bloodstream. Instead, they interact with cannabinoid receptors located in the skin, muscles, and nearby tissues.

These receptors are part of the body's **endocannabinoid system**, which plays a role in regulating pain, inflammation, and muscle tension.

When applied to tight or inflamed areas of the neck and shoulders, these creams may help reduce localized inflammation, relax chronically contracted muscles, and dampen nerve irritation in the surrounding tissues.

For patients who carry a constant band of tension across the upper trapezius muscles or the base of the skull, this local muscle relaxation can sometimes lower the background signal that feeds into migraine triggers.

The scientific evidence for topical cannabinoids is still evolving, but many pain specialists report that they can be useful for **localized musculoskeletal pain**, particularly in areas like the neck, shoulders, and upper back.

In practical terms, patients often apply these creams to the base of the skull, the upper trapezius muscles, the sides of the neck, or the upper back where tension tends to accumulate.

If chronic muscle tension in the neck is quietly feeding your migraine system, loosening those muscles may help turn down the volume of the trigger signal.

Medications Often Used for Neck-Driven Head Pain

When the neck is clearly part of the problem, doctors often combine topical treatments with medications that target inflammation, muscle spasm, and nerve irritation.

The goal is to calm all three parts of the problem at once. Anti-inflammatory drugs like **ibuprofen** or prescription NSAIDs such as **nabumetone** are frequently used to reduce inflammation in the cervical joints and surrounding soft tissue.

Muscle relaxers such as **methocarbamol** can help reduce the persistent muscle spasms that develop in the neck and upper shoulders when those muscles have been overworking for long periods of time.

And medications like **gabapentin**, which were originally developed to treat seizures, are now widely used to calm irritated nerve pathways and reduce neuropathic pain, including irritation involving the occipital nerves.

Each of these medications targets a slightly different part of the problem. NSAIDs reduce inflammation. Muscle relaxers calm the muscular tension that compresses nerves. Nerve-modulating medications reduce the sensitivity of the irritated nerves themselves.

When the neck is involved, treating all three layers of the system can sometimes dramatically reduce the frequency or intensity of headaches.

The Big Picture

If your headaches frequently begin with neck stiffness, soreness at the base of the skull, tenderness when pressing along the occipital nerves, or attacks triggered by posture, lifting, or cervical loading, then the neck may not simply be collateral damage from the migraine. It may be part of the cause.

In those cases, treating the cervical system directly becomes an important piece of the larger migraine strategy. Addressing neck inflammation, muscle tension, and nerve irritation can sometimes remove one of the sparks that lights the migraine fuse in the first place.

And if your neck is one of your triggers, turning down that signal can make the entire migraine system quieter.

The Trigeminocervical Complex:

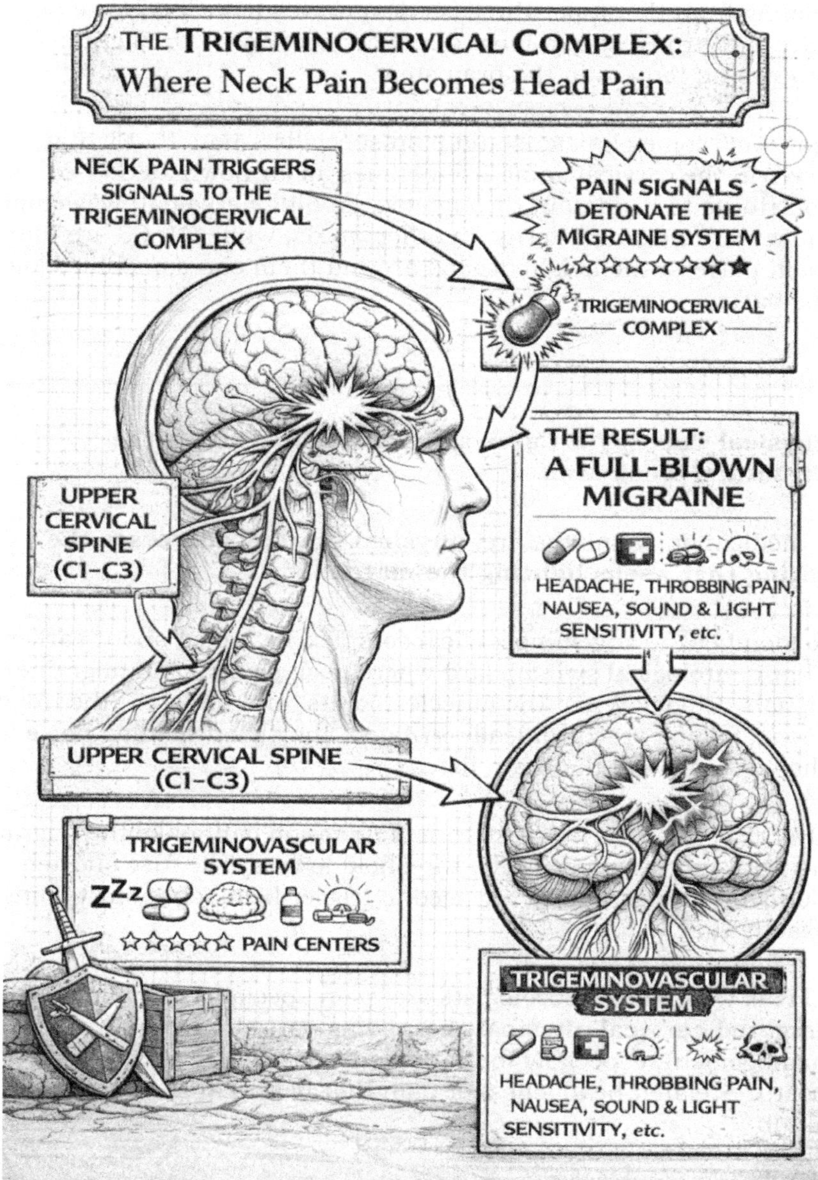

This image was created with the help of AI.

A Quick Anatomical Note:

Most descriptions of the trigeminocervical complex focus on signals coming from the upper three cervical nerves (C1–C3). These nerves have the strongest and most direct connections with migraine-processing centers in the brainstem.

However, some clinicians and pain specialists note that irritation lower in the cervical spine—sometimes as far down as C4—can still contribute to head pain through overlapping nerve pathways and muscular referral patterns. In other words, while C1–C3 are the main players, the neighborhood around them can sometimes join the party.

Physical Therapy & Cervical Stabilization: Fixing the Structural Weak Link

If medication calms the fire, **physical therapy addresses the wiring that keeps lighting the match**.

Remember the trigeminocervical complex we talked about earlier? That neurological switchboard where neck signals and migraine signals collide? When the muscles, joints, and nerves of the upper cervical spine are chronically irritated, they keep sending noise into that system. And the brain listens.

Over time, that constant stream of irritation can make the migraine network more sensitive. The threshold lowers. The fuse shortens. Suddenly things that never used to trigger headaches start doing exactly that.

This is why many neurologists and pain specialists now include **targeted cervical physical therapy** as part of migraine management, especially for patients who report neck stiffness, posture-related headaches, or pain that begins at the base of the skull.

The goal isn't just stretching a few tight muscles. The goal is **rebuilding stability in the entire cervical support system**.

Because here's the uncomfortable truth about the modern human spine: our necks were not designed for a world where we spend eight hours a day looking down at glowing rectangles.

Forward-head posture, rounded shoulders, and prolonged sitting gradually overload the small stabilizing muscles that support the cervical spine. Those muscles fatigue, larger muscles take over, and tension builds around the occipital nerves.

Eventually the system starts to complain. A good physical therapist trained in cervical disorders or headache medicine will usually focus on three core areas.

First is **postural correction**. This involves retraining how the head sits over the shoulders and how the upper spine supports that weight. Small adjustments here can dramatically reduce the mechanical stress placed on the upper cervical joints.

Second is **deep neck flexor strengthening**. These tiny muscles at the front of the neck act like the internal scaffolding that stabilizes the cervical spine. In many chronic headache sufferers, these muscles are weak or underactive, forcing the larger neck muscles to compensate and tighten.

Reactivating these deep stabilizers can take pressure off the irritated structures that feed the migraine pathways.

Third is **mobility work and soft tissue release**. Tight trapezius muscles, suboccipital muscles, and upper back tissues can compress nerves and restrict normal movement.

Carefully targeted stretching, manual therapy, and mobility exercises help restore normal motion and reduce nerve irritation.

The result is not instant magic. But over weeks and months, many patients notice something subtle but powerful: the baseline tension in their neck begins to drop. And when the neck quiets down, the migraine system often follows.

Some patients also benefit from **specific cervical stabilization programs**, which combine strengthening, posture training, and movement correction into a structured plan designed to reduce stress on the cervical spine long-term.

Think of it like reinforcing the foundation of a house. You can keep repainting the walls when cracks appear, but if the foundation is unstable, the cracks will keep coming back. Strengthen the foundation, and the entire structure becomes more resilient.

For migraine sufferers whose attacks consistently begin with neck stiffness, posture-related pain, or tenderness at the base of the skull, physical therapy is not just a supportive treatment. Sometimes it is **one of the missing pieces of the puzzle**.

A Final Note About the Neck

If neck pain is a dominant feature of your headaches, it is worth asking your doctor whether conditions such as **occipital neuralgia, cervicogenic headache, or cervical spine dysfunction** could be contributing to your attacks. These conditions frequently overlap with migraine, and they often require slightly different treatment strategies.

In other words, sometimes the migraine story doesn't start in the brain alone. Sometimes it starts a few inches lower.

Conclusion: Building Your Fortress, One Brick at a Time

We've just climbed the entire Ladder of Preventive Therapies, from the simple act of drinking water to injecting yourself with futuristic antibodies. It's a lot to process, and it can feel overwhelming. You might be tempted to try everything at once.

Don't.

Building a successful preventive strategy is a marathon, not a sprint. It is a slow, methodical process of trial, error, and patience. It often takes 2-3 months for a new preventive medication or supplement to show its full effect. Throwing everything at the wall at once won't tell you what's actually working.

The most effective way to build your fortress is one brick at a time, starting from the ground up, always in partnership with a doctor who listens to you.

Time for homework. And this one is simple: pick one thing.

Look at Tier 1. Which of those foundational bricks in your fortress is the most wobbly? Is it your sleep? Your stress levels? Your hydration? Choose the one that you know, deep down, you've been slacking on.

For the next 30 days, make that your singular focus. If it's sleep, you will go to bed and wake up at the exact same time every single day. No exceptions. If it's stress, you will schedule and complete a five-minute mindfulness meditation every single day. If it's hydration, that water bottle will become a new appendage you are never without.

Master one defense before you add another. A fortress built with one carefully placed brick at a time is infinitely stronger than one built with a hundred bricks thrown hastily in a pile.

You have your acute playbook for the fires that are burning now, and a long-term prevention strategy to keep future fires from starting. In the next section, PART IV: THRIVE, we shift gears. The hard science is behind you. Now we talk about something equally important: how to actually live well while managing this condition.

Chapter 8: Environmental Engineering

Hacking Your Habitat

Welcome to Part IV: THRIVE. You've graduated from basic training, learned to anticipate the enemy, and mastered your battle plans. You are no longer just surviving; you are fighting back, and you are winning.

But a warrior cannot live on the battlefield forever. Constantly fighting, defending, and reacting is exhausting. The ultimate victory isn't just winning the war; it's creating a life of peace so profound that many battles are never fought in the first place. This is where we shift from being soldiers to being architects.

This chapter is about Environmental Engineering. It's the art and science of "hacking your habitat"---methodically transforming your everyday surroundings from a potential trigger minefield into a personalized, migraine-proof sanctuary.

Let's be brutally honest: you cannot control the world. You cannot control the weather, the barometric pressure, or the fact that your company decided to install fluorescent lights that flicker with the intensity of a 1970s disco. But you can control your personal environment. You can control your bedroom, your office, and your digital spaces.

By systematically reducing the daily "trigger load" on your hypersensitive nervous system, you lower the water level in your migraine bucket (remember that from Chapter 4?). This means it takes a much bigger, more catastrophic combination of triggers to push you over the threshold into an attack. This isn't about living in a bubble; it's about being a damn smart engineer. It's about taking control of the variables you can influence, so you have more resilience to handle the ones you can't.

So, roll up your sleeves. We're about to become the ultimate life-hackers, redesigning our world one room at a time.

The Bedroom: Your Recovery Sanctum

Your bedroom is not just a place where you sleep. For a migraine warrior, it is your med bay, your recovery pod, your command center, and your panic room all in one. It is the single most important environment you can control. Optimizing your bedroom for deep, restorative sleep and acute-attack comfort is not a luxury; it is a non-negotiable part of your treatment plan. A poor night's sleep is one of the biggest, heaviest dominoes you can place in your trigger cascade. Our mission here is to remove that domino entirely.

Let's build your sleep sanctuary, one checklist at a time.

✓ The Blackout Protocol: Achieving True Darkness

Your brain's sleep-wake cycle is regulated by light. Even small amounts of light pollution---from streetlights, a neighbor's porch light, or the glaringly bright moon---can disrupt the production of melatonin, the hormone that tells your body it's time to sleep. For a migraine brain that's already hypersensitive to light (photophobia), this is even more critical.

- Blackout Curtains Are Non-Negotiable: Don't mess around with "room-darkening" flimsy nonsense. You need industrial-grade, soul-stealing, "is-it-day-or-night-I-genuinely-can't-tell" blackout curtains.
- Pro-Tip: For maximum effect, use a wrap-around curtain rod. This allows the curtain to curve back and touch the wall, eliminating that infuriating sliver of light that leaks from the sides.
- Budget Hack: If custom curtains aren't in the budget, you can buy blackout liners to clip onto the back of your existing curtains. Or, in a pinch, black construction paper or aluminum foil taped to the window works wonders. It's not pretty, but neither is a migraine.
- Eliminate Internal Light Pollution: The "enemy" isn't just outside. It's the tiny, blinking vampire lights from all your electronics.
- Cover or unplug the charging light on your phone, the power indicator on your TV, your digital alarm clock, and your Wi-Fi router. A small piece of electrical tape works perfectly.
- Invest in a high-quality, contoured sleep mask that doesn't put pressure on your eyes. This is your portable darkness, essential for travel or daytime naps.

✓ Temperature Control: The Cooler, The Better

Your body temperature naturally drops as you fall asleep. Keeping your room cool helps facilitate this process, leading to deeper, more restorative sleep. The ideal temperature range for sleep is generally between 60-67°F (15-19°C).

- A thermostat] Program Your Thermostat: If you have a programmable thermostat, set it to automatically cool down an hour before your bedtime. Let technology do the work.
- Create Airflow: A simple fan can help circulate air and keep you cool. The white noise it produces can also help mask other disruptive sounds.
- Mind the Humidity: A room that's too humid or too dry can disrupt sleep. A humidifier in the winter and a dehumidifier in the summer can help maintain a comfortable balance (aim for 40-50% humidity).

✓ Pillow Ergonomics: Protecting Your Neck

Remember our discussion of Occipital Neuralgia and cervicogenic headaches in Chapter 2? Your pillow is either your greatest ally or a secret saboteur in the fight against neck-related head pain. A pillow that's too high, too low, or too flimsy can put your cervical spine out of alignment, straining your neck muscles and irritating your occipital nerves all night long. Waking up with a stiff neck isn't just a bad start to the day; it's a potential migraine trigger.

Your Sleeping Position Dictates Your Pillow:

- Side Sleepers: You need a firmer, higher-loft pillow that fills the space between your ear and the mattress, keeping your head and neck in a straight line with your spine. Look for gusseted pillows that have extra fabric panels on the side to maintain their shape.
- Back Sleepers: You need a medium-loft, medium-firmness pillow. It should be just thick enough to support the natural curve of your neck without pushing your head too far forward. A cervical pillow with a built-in neck roll can be a game-changer.
- Stomach Sleepers: First of all, please stop. This is the worst position for your neck. But if you must, you need a very

thin, soft pillow, or no pillow at all, to avoid cranking your neck into an unnatural position.

- The "Wall Test": Not sure what height you need? Stand with your shoulder against a wall, in your natural sleeping posture. Measure the distance from your ear to the wall. That's roughly the loft (height) you need in a pillow if you're a side sleeper.

Pillow Materials:

Memory Foam: Conforms to your head and neck, providing excellent support. Can sometimes trap heat.

Latex: Bouncier and more breathable than memory foam, but also firm.

- Buckwheat: A personal favorite. These pillows are filled with buckwheat hulls and are incredibly adjustable. You can add or remove hulls to get the perfect height and firmness. They are also very breathable and supportive.
- Down/Feather: Luxuriously soft, but often lack the support needed to prevent neck strain unless they are extremely dense.

Your pillow is a critical piece of medical equipment. Invest in a good one and replace it every 1-2 years. It's cheaper than a lifetime of chiropractic appointments.

The Office: Your Productivity Bunker

For many of us, the modern office is a migraine-triggering torture chamber designed by someone who has clearly never had a headache in their life. The lighting is an affront to God and man, the noise level is a chaotic symphony of keyboard clatter and loud talkers, and the ergonomics seem purpose-built to create neck strain.

Whether you work in a corporate cubicle farm or a home office, it's time to transform your workspace from a source of pain into a productivity bunker. Your goal is to create an environment where you can do your best work without your brain staging a protest.

✓ Lighting Warfare: Banishing the Flicker

This is the biggest battle you will fight in the office. Standard-issue overhead fluorescent lighting is the arch-nemesis of the migraine brain, and for good reason.

- The Problem with Fluorescents: They don't just produce light; they produce a high-frequency, invisible flicker that your brain can detect even if your eyes can't. This constant, subliminal strobing is like torture for a hyper-excitable nervous system. They also emit a harsh, blue-spectrum light that is known to be particularly aggravating for photophobia.

Your Lighting Solution: You must become a ruthless advocate for better lighting.

- Kill the Overheads: If you can, turn off the fluorescent lights directly above your desk. This is your number one priority.
- Embrace Task Lighting: Use your own desk lamp with a warm-toned bulb instead. This puts you in control. Look for bulbs with a color temperature between 2700K and 3000K (this will be printed on the box). This range produces a softer, warmer, yellowish light that is much gentler on the eyes.
- Use Dimmers: Install a dimmer on your lamp so you can adjust the brightness throughout the day as your sensitivity levels change.
- Maximize Natural Light (Strategically): Position your desk so you can benefit from natural light from a window, but not so it creates a glare on your screen. Use blinds to control the intensity.

✓ The Sound of Silence: Managing Noise

An office is rarely quiet. Between phone calls, coworker chatter, and the relentless hum of the HVAC system, your auditory system is under constant low-grade assault. Your goal is to create a personal bubble of sound that you control.

- Invest in High-Quality Noise-Canceling Headphones: This is a non-negotiable investment. There are two types:
- Passive Noise Isolation: These are essentially high-tech earplugs (like over-ear studio headphones) that physically block sound.
- Active Noise Cancellation (ANC): These are the miracle workers. They use microphones to detect ambient noise and

then generate an opposing sound wave to cancel it out, creating a cone of near-silence. They are brilliant for tuning out low-frequency humming and chatter.

- Fight Fire with Fire (or, Noise with Noise): Sometimes, the most jarring sounds are the intermittent ones---a sudden laugh, a phone ringing. A white noise machine or an app on your phone (like myNoise or Noisli) can create a constant, predictable soundscape (like rain, a fan, or simple white noise) that masks these sudden interruptions, making your sound environment much less jarring.
- Communicate Your Needs: If you sit near a particularly loud colleague, it's okay to have a polite conversation. Try: "Hey, I'm really sensitive to noise because of my migraines. Would you mind taking longer calls in the conference room?"

✓ Ergonomic Engineering: Saving Your Neck

Remember how we talked about neck strain being a major domino that can topple into a migraine or Occipital Neuralgia attack? Your desk setup is either helping you or actively trying to sabotage your cervical spine. Let's fix it.

The Throne: Your chair is your foundation.

Ensure it has good lumbar support to keep your lower back in its natural curve.

Adjust the height so your feet are flat on the floor and your knees are at a roughly 90-degree angle.

- Your armrests should be positioned so your shoulders are relaxed, not hunched up by your ears.

The Monitor Position: This is the big one for preventing "tech neck."

- The top of your monitor should be at or just below eye level. If you have to look down at your screen (especially a laptop), you are putting immense strain on your neck muscles.
- Use a monitor stand or a stack of books to raise your screen to the proper height. If you use a laptop, get an external keyboard and mouse so you can raise the laptop screen while keeping your hands in a comfortable position.

Keyboard and Mouse Placement:

- Position them so your elbows are at a comfortable 90-degree angle and your wrists are straight, not bent up or down. This prevents shoulder and wrist strain that can travel up to your neck.
- The Micro-Break Protocol: Do not sit like a gargoyle for hours on end. Set a timer and follow the 20-20-20 rule: every 20 minutes, look at something 20 feet away for 20 seconds to give your eyes a break. Better yet, get up every 30-45 minutes for a quick stretch. Roll your shoulders, gently tuck your chin to your chest, and walk around for a minute. This is not slacking off; it is essential preventive maintenance for your body.

The Digital World: Taming the Pixels

Our screens are our windows to the world, but for a migraine brain, they can be portals to pain. The light, the flicker, and the constant focus they demand can be major triggers. It's time to tame these glowing rectangles.

✓ Screen Settings: Mastering Brightness and Contrast

The default settings on most devices are designed to look vibrant and eye-catching in a brightly lit store, which is the exact opposite of what you need.

- Brightness is Not Your Friend: Your screen should not be a light source. It should not illuminate your face in a dark room. A good rule of thumb is to match your screen's brightness to the ambient light in your room. It should be just bright enough to read comfortably, without squinting or feeling like you're staring into a headlight.
- Embrace the Dark Side: Dark Mode is one of the greatest gifts to migraine-kind. On your phone, your computer, and any app that supports it, switch to a dark background with light text. This drastically reduces the amount of light being blasted into your retinas and can significantly decrease eye strain and light sensitivity.

✓ Blue Light Warfare: Protecting Your Brain and Sleep

Blue light is a high-energy wavelength of light emitted by our screens. During the day, it's not terrible, but at night, it tricks our brain into thinking it's still daytime, which suppresses melatonin production and wrecks our sleep---a primary migraine defense.

Use Built-In Filters: Most modern operating systems have built-in blue light filters.

On Windows, it's called "Night light."

On Apple devices (Mac, iPhone, iPad), it's called "Night Shift."

- Set these to turn on automatically from sunset to sunrise. They will give your screen a warmer, amber tint that is much easier on the eyes and less disruptive to your sleep cycle.

Get Medical-Grade Glasses: The FL-41 Advantage:

- This is a pro-level hack. Not all "blue light blocking" glasses are created equal. Many just have a simple yellow tint. But FL-41 glasses are different. This is a specific, medical-grade tint, originally developed to reduce sensitivity in patients with fluorescent light-induced blepharospasm.
- The FL-41 tint is a very precise rosy-pink color that is specifically formulated to filter out the most painful wavelengths of blue and green light (around 480-520 nm) that are known to trigger the photophobia pathways in the migraine brain.
- They are more effective than standard blue blockers for reducing light sensitivity, both from screens and from harsh indoor lighting. If you are significantly light-sensitive, investing in a pair of indoor FL-41 glasses can be life-changing.

Chapter Eight Conclusion: You Are the Architect

You've just been handed the blueprints to build a safer, more comfortable world for yourself. We've engineered your bedroom for recovery, fortified your office for productivity, and tamed the harsh glare of the digital world.

It might seem like a lot. It might feel like you're retreating from the world, building a bubble to live inside. Reframe that thought. You are not building a bubble; you are building a bunker. You are creating a strategic home base from which you can operate with more strength and resilience. Every environmental tweak you make, every trigger you eliminate from your habitat, is one less domino in the chain reaction. It's one less splash of water in your migraine bucket.

This gives you more capacity, more resilience, to handle the things you can't control---the weather, the hormonal shifts, the stressful life events. You're not hiding. You're preparing.

Don't try to do everything at once. Just pick the single biggest offender in your environment right now and fix it this week:

Terrible office chair? Replace it. Flickering overhead fluorescent? Kill it and get a desk lamp. Lumpy pillow wrecking your neck? Order the cervical one tonight. Screen brightness at maximum? Turn it down and switch to dark mode. One fix. This week. Your brain will notice.

Start with one small, achievable victory. You don't have to overhaul your entire life by Friday. Swap one lightbulb, adjust one screen, replace one pillow. Then notice how it feels. These changes are cumulative, and they are quiet—but over weeks and months, they add up to a meaningfully different daily experience.

Now that we've engineered your external world, it's time to look inward. In the next chapter, we're going to tackle the most complex environment of all: the one between your ears. It's time to talk about your mind and mood.

Chapter 9: Mind & Mood

Taming the Anxiety Beast

We've engineered the bedroom, hacked the office, built the arsenal. So why is there still a little monster in the back of your mind whispering, "When's the next one gonna hit?"

Welcome, warrior, to the most complex and treacherous environment you'll ever have to navigate: the one between your ears.

A migraine attack is a physical event, but the fallout is emotional. The constant threat of the next attack, the isolation of canceling plans, the guilt of missing work, the frustration of feeling misunderstood---it all takes a toll. Living with a chronic, unpredictable condition is a recipe for anxiety and depression. It's not a sign of weakness; it's a sign that you're a human being with a nervous system that is, frankly, sick of this crap.

This chapter is about taming the beast of anxiety and mood that so often rides shotgun with migraine. We're not going to talk about "positive vibes only" or any of that toxic wellness nonsense. We're going to talk about practical, psychological self-defense. These are quick, effective, science-backed drills you can use to rewire your brain, interrupt the downward spirals, and reclaim your mental peace. Because you are more than your migraine, and it's time we proved it.

The Anxiety-Migraine Doom Loop: The Hamster Wheel from Hell

Let's dissect the most vicious cycle in the migraine universe. I call it the Anxiety-Migraine Doom Loop.

It looks like this:

- You have a bad migraine attack. It's brutal. It costs you a day of work, a family dinner, your will to live---you know the drill.
- You develop a fear of the next attack. Your brain, in a misguided attempt to protect you, goes on high alert. This isn't a conscious thought; it's a deep, primal fear. What will

the next one ruin? When will it strike? This state of hyper-vigilance is also known as anxiety.

- Anxiety causes stress. This constant state of worry and fear floods your body with stress hormones like cortisol. Your muscles tense up, your breathing gets shallow, and your heart rate climbs.
- Stress is a massive migraine trigger. As we know, stress hormones lower your migraine threshold, making your hyper-excitable brain even more likely to fire off an attack.

You get another migraine attack. The very thing you were afraid of has now been brought on by your fear.

- Your fear is reinforced. Your brain says, "See? I was right to be scared! This is horrible! I should be even more scared next time!"

And so the hamster wheel from hell spins faster and faster. The more you fear the attacks, the more you trigger them. The more you trigger them, the more you fear them.

If you've ever found yourself pre-emptively canceling plans for a fun event "just in case" you get a migraine, you're in the Doom Loop. If you feel a jolt of pure panic every time you feel a slight twinge in your neck, you're in the Doom Loop. If you spend your good days worrying about when the next bad day will come, congratulations, you've got a season pass to the shittiest theme park ride ever invented.

Breaking this cycle is paramount. It requires learning to unhook your thoughts and emotions from the physical reality of the pain. It's not easy, but it is possible. The following drills are your wire cutters.

Quick Drills: Your Mental Self-Defense Toolkit

You don't need a Ph.D. in psychology to start taking control of your thought patterns. You just need a few simple, powerful exercises that you can practice. We're borrowing from two of the most effective forms of therapy for chronic pain: Cognitive Behavioral Therapy (CBT) and Acceptance and Commitment Therapy (ACT).

CBT Quick Drills: Debugging Your Brain's Faulty Code

CBT is based on a simple premise: your thoughts, feelings, and behaviors are interconnected. Change the thought patterns, change how you feel. Think of it as debugging the faulty code your migraine installed in your brain.

Drill #1: Catch, Check, Change

This is the bread and butter of CBT. It's a simple, three-step process for dealing with Automatic Negative Thoughts (ANTs)---those nasty, unhelpful thoughts that pop into your head automatically when you're in pain or feeling anxious.

- Step 1: CATCH the Thought. The first step is to simply become aware of the ANT. Notice it without judgment. What story is your brain telling you right now?
- Example ANT: You're in the middle of an attack, and the thought screams, "This pain is never going to end. I can't handle this."
- Step 2: CHECK the Thought. Now, you become a detective. You put that thought on trial and examine the evidence for and against it. Ask yourself:
- Is this thought 100% true? Has any migraine I've ever had literally lasted forever? No.
- What's a more realistic outcome? Based on past experience, this attack will be excruciating for several hours or a day, and then it will end, and I will recover.
- Is this thought helping me right now? No, it's just adding panic and suffering on top of my pain.
- Step 3: CHANGE the Thought. You don't have to change it to something ridiculously positive. We're not aiming for "I love my migraine!" That's delusional. We're aiming for something balanced and realistic.
- Example Changed Thought: "This pain is excruciating right now, and I hate it. But I have survived every single migraine I've had before this one, and I will survive this one too. This is temporary. My only job right now is to rest and use my tools."

This simple reframing doesn't make the pain go away. Nothing does. But what it does do is remove the second layer of suffering---the panic, the catastrophizing, the terror---that makes the physical pain so much worse.

MINI-CASE STORY #1: SARAH'S SHIFT

Sarah, a 34-year-old graphic designer, found that her panic during a migraine attack was almost as debilitating as the pain. Her go-to thought was always, "I'm going to lose my job if this keeps happening." During her next attack, she decided to try "Catch, Check, Change."

Catch: She noticed the thought: "I'm going to get fired." Check: She asked herself for evidence. "Has my boss ever threatened me? No. Have I communicated my condition and requested accommodations? Yes. Has my work quality suffered overall? No, just my attendance on bad days." The evidence didn't support the catastrophic thought. Change: She reframed it: "My boss knows I have a medical condition. This attack is forcing me to take a sick day, which is what sick days are for. I will communicate professionally and make up the work when I can. I am not going to get fired over this."

Sarah said that while the pain was still a 9/10, her suffering dropped to a 5/10. She was able to rest without the added layer of terror about her career, which she felt helped her recover faster.

ACT Quick Drills: Learning to Surf the Waves

Acceptance and Commitment Therapy has a different, but equally powerful, approach. ACT isn't about changing your thoughts; it's about changing your relationship to your thoughts. It teaches you that thoughts are just... thoughts. They are not orders. They are not facts. They are just words popping up in your head. You don't have to believe them or fight them. You can just notice them, unhook from them, and then commit to acting in a way that aligns with your values (like being a person who takes care of themselves).

If CBT is debugging the code, ACT is realizing you're not the computer; you're the person sitting at the keyboard. You can choose which programs to run.

Drill #2: Defusion --- Unhooking from Your Thoughts

Defusion is the art of creating distance between you and your thoughts, so you can see them for what they are: temporary mental events.

- The "I'm Having the Thought That..." Technique: This is the simplest and most profound defusion trick. When a painful thought arises, just add the phrase "I'm having the thought that..." to the beginning of it.

Instead of: "I am a terrible mother because this migraine is making me miss my son's school play."

Try: "I'm having the thought that I am a terrible mother because this migraine is making me miss my son's school play."

- Can you feel the difference? In the first sentence, you are a terrible mother. It's an identity. In the second, you are a person who is observing a thought. The thought is just an event happening in your mind. It's not you. This tiny linguistic shift creates just enough space for you to breathe and not get swept away by the current of self-criticism.
- The "Silly Voice" Technique: This sounds ridiculous, but it works. Take your most painful, scary thought, and say it out loud in the voice of a cartoon character.
- Imagine Bugs Bunny saying, "Ehhh, what's up, doc? This migraine is gonna last forever and ruin your life!"
- It's impossible to take a thought seriously when it sounds that absurd. This technique highlights the true nature of thoughts: they are just words, and we can choose not to give them power.

Drill #3: The Anchor --- Grounding Yourself in Reality

When you're spiraling in a vortex of pain, anxiety, or catastrophic thoughts, your mind is untethered from the present moment. It's either worrying about a future that hasn't happened or regretting a past you can't change. Grounding is the practice of dropping an anchor into the here and now. It pulls you out of the storm in your head and back into the physical reality of your body and your environment.

This is the 5-4-3-2-1 Grounding Technique. It's simple, it's fast, and you can do it anywhere, even while lying in your migraine cave.

- Step 1: NOTICE FIVE THINGS YOU CAN SEE. Look around you and silently name five things. Don't just list them; notice a detail about each one. "I see the crease on my grey blanket. I see the shadow my water bottle is casting. I see a speck of dust on the floor. I see the grain of wood on my nightstand. I see the light under the door." This forces your brain to engage with your sense of sight in a neutral, observational way.

- Step 2: NOTICE FOUR THINGS YOU CAN FEEL. Bring your awareness to the physical sensations of touch. "I can feel the soft texture of my pillowcase against my cheek. I can feel the weight of my cat sleeping on my legs. I can feel the cool air from the fan on my skin. I can feel the tension in my shoulders."
- Step 3: NOTICE THREE THINGS YOU CAN HEAR. Listen closely. What are the sounds in your environment? "I can hear the hum of the air purifier. I can hear the distant sound of traffic outside. I can hear my own breathing."
- Step 4: NOTICE TWO THINGS YOU CAN SMELL. This one can be tricky, but try. "I can smell the faint scent of the lavender pillow spray I used earlier. I can smell the clean scent of my laundry detergent on my sheets."
- Step 5: NOTICE ONE THING YOU CAN TASTE. What is the taste in your mouth right now? "I can taste the lingering flavor of the ginger tea I just sipped."

By the time you get to the end of this exercise, you've successfully pulled your brain out of the abstract world of worry and anchored it firmly in the present moment. You haven't solved the migraine, but you've interrupted the panic, which is a massive victory.

MINI-CASE STORY #2: BEN'S ANCHOR

Ben's biggest fear was his visual auras. The moment the shimmering lights started, his heart would pound, and he'd spiral into a panic attack, convinced he was having a stroke, even though he'd been through it a hundred times. His therapist taught him the 5-4-3-2-1 technique.

The next time an aura began, as the zig-zag lines started to creep across his vision, he immediately started the drill. "I see my keyboard. I see the coffee stain on my mousepad. I see the photo of my dog..." By the time he got to "I can feel the smooth plastic of my chair's armrest," he noticed his breathing had slowed. The aura was still there, and he knew the pain was coming, but the terror was gone. He was just a man, sitting in a chair, observing a weird neurological event. It allowed him to stay calm enough to take his rescue medication and calmly inform his wife, "The light show has started. Time to retreat."

The Guilt-Spiral Interrupt Protocol: Your 3-Step Off-Ramp

And now, for the most insidious emotional enemy of all: guilt. Migraine guilt is a special kind of poison. It's the feeling that you are unreliable, a burden, a failure for having a body that doesn't cooperate. It whispers that you've let down your partner, your kids, your friends, your boss. If the Anxiety Doom Loop is a hamster wheel, the Guilt Spiral is a toilet bowl, circling down into a sewer of self-blame.

It's time to install an emergency flush-interrupt. This is a simple, 3-step protocol to stop that spiral in its tracks.

Step 1: NOTICE & NAME ("The Acknowledgment")

- The moment you feel that familiar, sinking feeling of guilt, your first job is simply to notice it and name it. Don't fight it, don't ignore it. Just say to yourself, "Ah, there it is. I am feeling guilt right now."
- Naming the emotion separates you from it. You are not "guilty." You are a person experiencing the feeling of guilt. This creates a small but crucial space between you and the emotion.

Step 2: APPLY LOGIC & EVIDENCE ("The Reality Check")

- Now, you cross-examine that feeling. Guilt is only a valid emotion if you have done something intentionally wrong. Put your guilt on the witness stand and ask it some hard questions:
- "Did I choose to have a neurological condition?" (No.)
- "Did I wake up this morning and think, 'I would love to develop excruciating head pain and cancel my plans'?" (Definitely not.)
- "Am I intentionally trying to harm or inconvenience the people I love?" (Of course not.)
- The evidence is clear: Your condition is not your fault. Therefore, the guilt is not based in logic. It's an irrational emotional response to a biological problem.

Step 3: PRACTICE RADICAL SELF-COMPASSION ("The Reframe")

- This is the final and most important step. You actively replace the voice of guilt with the voice of a kind, compassionate friend. Imagine what you would say to a best friend who was in your exact situation. You would never say, "You're so lazy and unreliable for getting sick." You would say something loving. So say that to yourself.
- Example Reframe: "This is not my fault. This is my biology. It is not only okay for me to rest and take care of myself right now, it is my absolute responsibility. The people who love me will understand, and my true friends would want me to prioritize my health. I am doing the best I can with a difficult situation."

This three-step protocol is your off-ramp from the highway to self-loathing. Practice it every single time you feel the guilt creeping in. It will feel unnatural at first, but with repetition, you will build new neural pathways. You will train your brain to default to compassion instead of condemnation.

MINI-CASE STORY #3: MARIA'S INTERRUPT

Maria had to miss her nephew's 5th birthday party because of a severe migraine. The guilt was eating her alive. She pictured her sister being disappointed and her nephew being sad. She started down the spiral: "I'm a terrible aunt. I'm so unreliable. They're all going to stop inviting me to things."

Then she remembered the protocol. Notice & Name: "Okay. This is guilt. I feel heavy and awful." Apply Logic: "Did I want to miss the party? No, I was looking forward to it all week. Can I control the timing of my attacks? No." Practice Self-Compassion: She told herself, "A good aunt is one who loves her nephew, not just one who shows up to every party. A good sister is one who takes care of her health so she can be there in the long run. I will call him tomorrow when I feel better and send him his gift."

By interrupting the spiral, Maria was able to focus on recovery instead of self-flagellation. The next day, she had a lovely video call with her nephew, who was just excited to show her his new toys. Her sister wasn't mad at all; she was just worried. The catastrophe Maria had imagined was entirely in her head.

ACTION BOX: Mindfulness in 60 Seconds

Need to interrupt a stress or panic spiral RIGHT NOW? Use this simple Box Breathing exercise. You can do it anywhere---at your desk, in your car, in the bathroom at a party. It works by regulating your breath, which sends a direct signal to your vagus nerve to calm your entire nervous system down.

1. **Breathe in slowly through your nose for a count of 4. (Feel your belly expand).**
2. **Hold your breath gently for a count of 4. (Don't clench).**
3. **Breathe out slowly through your mouth for a count of 4. (Gently empty your lungs).**
4. **Hold your breath at the bottom for a count of 4.**
5. **Repeat the cycle for 60 seconds, or as long as you need.**

♥□ A Note to Your Inner Circle: You're Carrying Something Heavy Too

This section is written directly for the partners, parents, friends, siblings, and anyone else who loves someone with chronic migraines. If that's you, please read this. It was written for you.

You don't have a migraine. But you live with one.

You've rearranged plans, managed the house alone during attacks, fielded disappointed calls from people who don't understand why your person had to cancel again. You've tiptoed through darkened rooms, kept kids quiet, swallowed your frustration when a rare good evening ended abruptly because of a warning sign only they can feel. You've been supportive and patient and loving, sometimes while quietly carrying your own grief about what this condition has cost you both.

Nobody wrote a chapter for you. We're fixing that.

What you might be feeling is real, and it has a name.

Compassion fatigue is a recognized psychological phenomenon that affects caregivers and close supporters of people with chronic illness. It doesn't mean you love your person less. It doesn't mean you're selfish or a bad partner. It means you've been pouring from your cup for a long time, and nobody reminded you to refill it.

The symptoms are real: exhaustion that doesn't improve with rest, growing resentment or emotional numbness, a sense of helplessness or hopelessness about whether things will ever improve, feeling like your own needs have become invisible or irrelevant. Sometimes a low-grade grief for the relationship or the life you imagined, or for plans that keep getting canceled and adventures you haven't taken yet.

These are not signs of failure. They are signs that you are human, and that caring deeply about someone in chronic pain is its own kind of hard.

What actually helps -- for you, not just for them:

You are allowed to have needs. You are allowed to say, "This week was hard for me too." You are allowed to grieve canceled plans and interrupted moments without immediately qualifying it with "but I know it's not their fault." Both things can be true at the same time: it's not their fault, and it still hurts.

Find someone outside the relationship to talk to -- a friend, a therapist, a support group for partners of people with chronic illness. Not to complain about your person, but to be witnessed in your own experience. You deserve that witness. You cannot be a good support system if you are running on empty and pretending you're not.

Be honest with your person, gently, about where you are. Chronic illness partnerships thrive when both people feel seen, not when one person silently martyrs themselves while the other assumes everything is fine. Your honesty is not a burden -- it's an invitation to face this together instead of parallel to each other.

What your person probably wants you to know, but may not know how to say:

They see what it costs you. The guilt they carry about the impact on your life is often as heavy as anything else they carry. When they seem withdrawn or distant in their good moments, it's sometimes because they're bracing for the next bad one, or because they've spent so long apologizing that they don't know how to just be normal with you anymore.

The single most healing thing you can do -- for them and for you -- is to occasionally be explicitly okay. Tell them you're in this. Tell them you love them and you're not going anywhere. Tell them that even the difficult version of this life is one you'd choose. You don't have to perform optimism. Just honesty. Just presence.

You are not a caregiver. You are a person who loves someone with a chronic condition. That is its own identity, and it deserves its own care.

Chapter Nine Conclusion: You Are Not Your Thoughts

The battle for your mind is just as important as the battle for your head. The pain of a migraine is unavoidable, but the suffering that comes from anxiety, panic, and guilt is optional. It's a second layer of misery that you do not have to endure.

You cannot stop your brain from generating thoughts. It's a thought machine; that's its job. It will continue to serve up unhelpful, catastrophic, and self-critical garbage, especially when you're in a vulnerable state. Your power lies not in stopping the thoughts, but in changing your relationship to them.

You can notice them without believing them. You can challenge them with evidence. You can create distance from them. You can anchor yourself in the present moment when they try to pull you into a storm. You are the sky, not the weather. The thoughts are just clouds passing through.

So here is your actionable mission for this chapter. Don't try to become a Zen master overnight. Just pick one of the drills we've talked about.

Is it Catch, Check, Change?

Is it the 5-4-3-2-1 Grounding technique?

Is it the Guilt-Spiral Interrupt?

Choose the one that resonates most with you. Write it on a sticky note. Put it on your bathroom mirror or your computer monitor. Keep it in your back pocket like a secret weapon. The next time you feel that familiar dread, panic, or self-blame bubbling up, deploy it. Don't worry about doing it perfectly. Just try.

You don’t have to master this overnight. You just have to start noticing. That is the first move, and it is enough.

Now that you have the tools to start engineering your internal world, it's time to take on the external one. In the next chapter, we'll get tactical about navigating the complexities of work, school, and relationships when you're living with a chaotic brain.

Chapter 10: Your Life Support

Work, School & Relationships

You've learned to decode your brain, dodge the dominoes, and fight back with an arsenal. But you don't live in a vacuum. You live in a world of bosses, deadlines, final exams, and friends who want brunch in offensively bright restaurants.

Life doesn't stop when a migraine hits. The bills keep coming, the kids still need to be fed, and your boss probably thinks your "bad headache" should be no match for the quarterly earnings report.

This chapter is your diplomatic training manual for navigating work, school, and relationships when your brain is a chaotic, unreliable narrator.

The goal isn't survival—it's teaching the people in your life to be part of your support crew instead of another trigger. Let's get tactical.

At Work: How to Slay Deadlines, Not Your Career

Having a conversation with your boss about a chronic, invisible illness is about as appealing as a root canal during a lightning storm. But hiding your condition and trying to "power through" is a guaranteed recipe for burnout.

Advocating for yourself in the workplace is not a sign of weakness; it is a sign of professional maturity. It shows that you understand your body, you are serious about managing your health, and you are committed to finding a way to perform your job effectively in the long term.

Talking to HR & Your Boss: The Strategic Disclosure

You don't have to tell everyone in the office about your medical history. But telling your direct manager and/or Human Resources is a strategic move that protects you and sets you up for success.

- Know Your Rights (The Legal Basics): Before you say a word, know where you stand. In the United States, migraine can be considered a disability under the Americans with Disabilities Act (ADA). This is a huge deal. It means that if you work for a company with 15 or more employees, you are legally entitled to "reasonable accommodations"---modifications to your job or work environment that allow you to perform your essential duties. This isn't your company doing you a favor; it's them following the law. (If you live outside the US, research your country's specific disability and employment laws).

The Conversation:

- Timing is Everything: Don't have this conversation in the middle of a crisis. Schedule a private meeting when you and your manager are calm and not rushed.
- Be Confident and Solution-Oriented: You are not coming to them with a problem; you are coming to them as a proactive employee with a plan. Frame it as, "I want to discuss how I can continue to do my best work while managing a recurring medical condition."
- Keep it Professional: You don't need to share the gory details of your worst attack. Keep the explanation concise and focused on how it impacts your work. For example: "I have a diagnosed neurological condition called migraine. The attacks are unpredictable and can temporarily cause symptoms like severe pain and sensitivity to light and sound, which can make it difficult to work at my desk."

The Golden Ticket: Your Template for Requesting Accommodations

This is where you formalize your request. An email creates a paper trail and shows that you are taking this process seriously. It should be sent to your direct manager and, if appropriate, an HR representative. Feel free to copy, paste, and customize this bad boy.

TOOL: TEMPLATE EMAIL FOR HR ACCOMMODATIONS

Subject: Request for Reasonable Accommodations

Dear [Manager's Name] and/or [HR Representative's Name],

This email is to formally request reasonable accommodations for a medical condition as provided for under the Americans with Disabilities Act (ADA).

I have a diagnosed neurological condition, Chronic Migraine, which can cause debilitating symptoms including severe head pain, nausea, and extreme sensitivity to light and sound. These symptoms, while temporary, can impact my ability to work effectively in the standard office environment.

I am committed to performing all of my essential job functions at a high level. To help me manage my condition and maintain my productivity, I am requesting the following accommodations:

- Lighting Adjustments: Permission to turn off the overhead fluorescent lighting at my workstation and use my own lamp with a non-flickering, warm-toned bulb.
- Flexible Scheduling/Telework: The ability to work from home on days when I am experiencing a severe migraine attack but am still capable of working.
- Screen Filters: Permission to use a privacy filter or blue-light-blocking filter on my computer monitor to reduce glare.
- Unscheduled Breaks: The ability to take short, infrequent breaks in a quiet area (such as a wellness room or empty office) to manage acute symptoms when they arise.

I believe these accommodations will allow me to manage my condition effectively and continue to be a productive member of our team. I am happy to provide medical documentation from my physician to support this request and am open to discussing any alternative accommodations that may also be effective.

Thank you for your time and consideration.

Sincerely,

[Your Name]

- The Snarky Take: This email is your secret weapon. It's polite, professional, and dripping with just the right amount of "I know my rights." It's the corporate equivalent of saying, "I'd prefer not to sue you, but let's not find out what happens if you ignore this, okay?"

At School: Acing Your Grades Without Acing Your Health

The academic world is it's own special kind of migraine hell. Long study hours, inconsistent sleep schedules, fluorescent-lit libraries, and the stress of exams create a perfect storm of triggers. Whether you are a student with migraine or the parent of one, advocating for academic modifications is not about getting an "easy pass"---it's about leveling the playing field so that a biological condition doesn't derail an education.

Getting Ahead of the Problem

The key to success is being proactive. Don't wait until you've missed a major exam to have a conversation.

- For College Students: Register with the Disability Services or Accessibility Office at the beginning of the semester. This is your campus HR. They are the experts in academic accommodations. They will review your medical documentation and create an official letter of accommodation that you can then give to your professors. This takes the burden of negotiation off your shoulders.
- For Parents of Younger Students: Schedule a meeting with your child's teacher, school counselor, and school nurse before the school year starts, or as soon as a diagnosis is made. Frame the conversation around collaboration: "We want to partner with you to ensure [Child's Name] can succeed academically while managing their health."

The Ultimate Checklist for a Migraine-Friendly Education

You can use this list as a starting point for discussions with teachers, professors, or disability services staff. Pick the ones that are most relevant to your (or your child's) needs.

TOOL: CHECKLIST OF POTENTIAL CLASSROOM MODIFICATIONS

[ ] Environmental Accommodations:

Preferential Seating: A seat away from windows, bright lights, or other known environmental triggers.

Lighting Adjustments: Permission to wear tinted glasses (such as FL-41s) or a brimmed hat in the classroom.

- Scent-Aware Classroom: A request for the classroom to be a "scent-free" or "scent-aware" zone, especially in labs with strong chemicals.

[ ] Attendance & Breaks:

- Excused Absences/Tardies: A flexible attendance policy for absences due to documented severe migraine attacks, without academic penalty.
- Access to a Quiet Rest Area: Permission to go to the nurse's office or a designated quiet room to rest and take medication at the onset of an attack.

[ ] **Assignments & Deadlines:**

- Flexible Deadlines: The ability to request a pre-arranged extension on major assignments when a migraine attack interferes with the ability to complete them on time.
- Advance Notice for Major Projects: Receiving syllabi and major project deadlines as early as possible to allow for advance planning around potential migraine days.

[ ] **Testing Accommodations:**

Extended Time: Allowing extra time (e.g., time-and-a-half) on tests and exams to account for brain fog or pain.

- Testing in a Separate, Quiet Location: Taking exams in a distraction-free and quiet environment to minimize sensory triggers.

Breaks During Exams: Permission to take short breaks during long exams as needed.

[ ] **In-Class Support:**

Note-Taking Assistance: Access to a peer's or instructor's notes for classes missed due to a migraine.

- Use of Technology: Permission to use a laptop for note-taking to reduce eye strain from looking up and down, or to use screen-reading software.

In Relationships: How to Explain Your Needs Without Sounding Like a Broken Record

Now we enter the most personal arena of all: your relationships. This is your life support, your inner circle, the people whose love and understanding can feel like the most powerful medicine in the world... or whose skepticism and misunderstanding can feel like another trigger entirely.

The core challenge in any relationship, when you're a migraine warrior, is communication. How do you explain the invisible? How do you articulate the unpredictable? How many times can you say, "I have a migraine," before you start to feel like a broken record, and you worry that your loved ones hear it as, "I'm making another excuse"?

The secret is to shift from being a reporter of your pain to being a collaborator in your own care. It's not just about announcing an attack; it's about proactively teaching the people you love how to be on your team.

Communicating with Your Romantic Partner: Us vs. The Migraine

Your partner sees it all: the good days, the bad days, and the can't-move-from-the-darkened-room days. The goal is to transform them from a worried bystander into your trusted second-in-command.

- Have "The Talk" (During Peacetime): Do not try to have a deep, meaningful conversation about your condition in the middle of an attack. It will not go well. Schedule a time when you are both calm and feeling good. This is a strategy meeting for "Team You."
- Explain Your "Tells": Let them know what your prodrome symptoms are. "Hey, if you ever see me yawning uncontrollably or suddenly craving salt, that's a yellow alert. It means an attack might be coming, and I need to start my preventive protocol."
- Create an Action Plan Together: What is their role during Code Red? Do you want them to bring you an ice pack? Make sure your meds and water are by the bed? Run interference with the kids? Write it down together. This gives them a clear, helpful job, which can alleviate their feeling of helplessness.
- Teach Them Your Language: Explain what you mean when you say certain things. "When I say 'the lights are too bright,' I don't mean they're a little annoying. I mean they feel like physical daggers in my eyeballs."

The Ultimate Script for a Partner:

"I want us to be a team against this. When I have an attack, I'm not pushing you away; I'm retreating from the pain. The single most helpful thing you can do is trust that I know what my body needs, which is usually just darkness and silence. Knowing you're handling things on the outside so I can recover on the inside is the greatest support you can give me. We're in this together: us against the migraine."

Communicating with Friends: Preserving Your Social Lifeline

Friendships can be one of the first casualties of chronic migraine. The constant canceling of plans can lead to you feeling guilty and your friends feeling blown off. Proactive communication is the only way to prevent this.

Educate Your Core Crew: Get your best friends together for a coffee (on a good day) and give them the short version.

"Hey guys, I want to be real with you about my migraines. They are a neurological condition, and they're super unpredictable. It means that sometimes, I have to bail on our plans at the last minute. Please know that when I do, I am absolutely gutted. It has nothing to do with not wanting to see you. It's just me needing to deal with a medical event. Your understanding means the world to me."

- Become the Planner: Instead of always reacting to invitations to loud bars or crowded venues, take the lead. Be the one to suggest migraine-friendly activities. "Hey, instead of the club on Friday, what if we did a bonfire at the beach?" or "Let's skip the noisy brunch spot and do a potluck at my place." This shows you are invested in the friendship, but you're doing it on terms that won't land you in a dark room for two days.

Communicating with Family: Navigating History and "Helpful" Advice

Oh, family. The source of our greatest comfort and, sometimes, our most infuriating advice. Dealing with family, especially older relatives who may come from a "just tough it out" generation, requires a special kind of diplomatic skill.

- For the Skeptic: For the family member who still thinks it's "just a headache," don't argue. State facts. "Migraine is recognized by the World Health Organization as one of the most disabling neurological diseases in the world. My neurologist and I are treating it as the serious medical condition it is." End of discussion. You don't need to win the debate; you just need to state your reality.

- For the "Advisor": This is the loved one who is constantly sending you articles about a new celery juice cleanse or asking, "Have you tried giving up gluten? My friend's cousin did, and..." This comes from a place of love, but it's exhausting.

The Script:

"Aunt Karen, I know you're only suggesting this because you care about me, and I truly appreciate that. It means a lot. My specialist and I have a very comprehensive medical plan that we're working on, and for now, I need to focus on that to see if it works. But thank you for thinking of me."

- Why it Works: It validates their good intentions ("I know you care"), creates a firm boundary ("My doctor and I have a plan"), and ends with gratitude. It's polite, loving, and a complete shutdown.

Your relationships are your life support. Investing the time to teach people how to be there for you is one of the most important preventive strategies you can ever undertake. And to make it easier, here's a tool you can literally hand them.

TOOL: A FAQ FOR YOUR CAREGIVER, PARTNER, OR ANYONE WHO LOVES YOU

(A Note to the Reader: Feel free to screenshot this, print it out, or email it to the people who are on your team. Sometimes it's easier to let the book do the talking.)

1. So, what is a migraine really? Is it just a bad headache?

Think of it less like a headache and more like a temporary, painful "computer crash" for the brain. It's a neurological event. During an attack, the brain's electrical systems go haywire, causing not just severe pain, but often a whole host of other symptoms like nausea, extreme sensitivity to light and sound, dizziness, and even trouble speaking. It's a full-body experience that is completely incapacitating.

2. What should I do (and what should I absolutely NOT do) when you're having an attack?

This is the most important question, and thank you for asking.

- DO: Ask quietly, "Is there anything I can get you?" The answer will probably be their medication, a glass of water, or an ice pack.

DO: Help create a "migraine cave." Dim the lights, turn off the TV, close the door. Silence and darkness are medicine.

DO: Offer to take a task off their plate. "Don't worry about dinner, I've got it."

DON'T: Ask a million questions. Their brain is being assaulted, and processing information is difficult and painful.

- DON'T: Suggest remedies. Now is not the time to bring up that article you saw about a new supplement. Trust that they are following their medical plan.
- DON'T: Make them feel guilty. Never say things like, "Again?" or "Are you sure you're not just tired?" The guilt is already immense; please don't add to it.

3. You cancel plans a lot. Does that mean you don't want to see me?

It means the exact opposite. When a migraine warrior has to cancel, it is heartbreaking. We were likely looking forward to that plan as a bright spot in a difficult week. Canceling is a last resort, done because the physical reality of the attack makes it impossible to function. It has absolutely nothing to do with our feelings for you. The best response is always, "I'm so sorry you're feeling awful. Don't worry about it at all. Let's reschedule when you're feeling better." That simple act of understanding is a massive gift.

4. I feel so helpless watching you suffer. What can I actually do to help?

Your understanding is the single most helpful thing you can offer. But if you want a practical job, here it is: be the guardian of the peace. Run interference. Keep the house quiet, tell the kids it's time for a quiet activity, and handle whatever life-admin task needs handling so the person suffering can fully retreat and recover. You aren't helpless; you are their shield. By taking on the world for a little while, you are giving them the space they need to heal. And that is everything.

📋 Quick Guide Cards: How to Support Someone with Migraine

(Cut these out. Screenshot them. Forward them. Tape them to the fridge. These are for the people in your corner who want to help but aren't sure how. Different roles, different responsibilities -- same team.)

🏠 QUICK GUIDE: For Partners & Spouses

Your role: Trusted second-in-command. You're not the nurse -- you're the CO.

When an attack starts:

- Create the migraine cave without being asked: dim lights, close door, lower TV volume.
- Offer one quiet question: "Do you need anything?" Then let them lead.
- Handle the household -- meals, kids, noise, incoming communications. Run the outside world so they can disappear inside.

What NOT to do:

- Don't ask a stream of questions. Their brain is struggling to process.
- Don't suggest home remedies or new supplements. They have a medical plan.
- Don't take the retreat personally. It's the migraine they're fleeing, not you.

On good days:

- Ask how you can best support them -- not during an attack, but between them.
- Notice the prodrome signs they've described and give a quiet heads-up: "Hey, you seem a bit off. Everything okay?"
- Remember you're allowed to have needs too. Speak up. A strong partnership talks about both sides.

👨‍👩‍👦 QUICK GUIDE: For Parents & Adult Children

Your role: Protector of their energy. Reduce the load; don't add to it.

When an attack starts:

- Take over immediately. Food, logistics, communication with others -- it's yours now.
- Protect their space. Keep younger siblings or household members quiet and occupied.
- Don't hover. They know you love them. What they need is space, not supervision.

What NOT to do:

- Don't share stories of "when you had headaches and pushed through." This is different.
- Don't question whether it's "really that bad." It is.
- Don't offer remedies unless they've asked. Chances are they've tried them all.

On good days:

- Check in warmly, not medically. Ask how life is going, not just how their head is.
- Celebrate the good days without projecting anxiety onto them about the next bad one.
- If they're navigating the healthcare system, offer to help -- driving to appointments, taking notes, being a second set of ears in the room.

👫 QUICK GUIDE: For Friends

Your role: The no-drama anchor. You make normal feel possible.

When they cancel:

- Your response matters more than you know. Say: "No worries at all -- let's reschedule. Rest up." That's it. No guilt. No "again?" No long silence.
- Don't post a bunch of fun photos from the night they missed. Give it a day.
- Check in the next day with something light: "Hope you're feeling better. Thinking of you."

When they're struggling:

- You don't need to fix anything. You just need to show up consistently.
- Suggest migraine-friendly hangouts: quiet dinners at home, a walk in the park, movie nights with dimmable lights. You keep the friendship alive; they'll love you for it.
- Don't disappear because plans keep changing. Chronic illness is lonely enough without losing friends too.

On good days:

- Be fully present. These are the days they've been waiting for.
- Don't bring up the condition unless they do. Give them a break from being the sick person.

□💼 QUICK GUIDE: For Managers & Employers

Your role: Informed ally. Flexibility is not charity -- it's good management.

What you need to know:

- Migraine is a neurological condition, not an attitude problem or a preference.
- It is recognized as a potential disability under the ADA (and equivalent laws internationally). Reasonable accommodations are a legal baseline, not a favor.
- Employees with migraine are often among the most motivated and conscientious workers precisely because they've had to fight so hard to stay functional.

What actually helps:

- Flexible remote work options on high-symptom days dramatically reduce both sick days and presenteeism (showing up and underperforming).
- Lighting accommodations are inexpensive and impactful -- a personal desk lamp can make a significant difference.
- A brief, private check-in conversation goes further than any HR policy. Ask what support looks like for them specifically.

What makes things worse:

- Skepticism about invisible symptoms. You don't need to see the pain to acknowledge it's real.

- Stigma or frustration expressed in the moment. They already feel guilty; your reaction shapes whether they'll communicate proactively next time or just call in sick with no explanation.
- Requiring detailed medical disclosures beyond what's legally necessary.

🍎 QUICK GUIDE: For Teachers & School Staff

Your role: Academic safety net. The goal is access, not advantage.

What you need to know:

- A student with migraine is not seeking an easy pass. They are trying to learn despite a biological obstacle.
- The invisible nature of migraine means attacks can hit mid-class, mid-exam, or mid-week without warning. This is not drama or avoidance -- it's neurological reality.
- Missed class time during an attack is recovery time, not leisure time.

What actually helps:

- A quiet space to retreat when an attack begins -- nurse's office, empty room, hallway with a pass.
- Flexible deadlines communicated in advance rather than negotiated in crisis.
- Access to notes or recordings for missed class time.
- Letting the student or parent proactively brief you at the start of term, so the first conversation isn't happening at the worst moment.

What makes things worse:

- Public check-ins during an attack. Privacy matters.
- Attendance penalties applied without acknowledgment of documented medical events.
- Skepticism. If a student says they're experiencing symptoms, believe them.

Conclusion: Communication is Your Superpower

You cannot control when a migraine strikes. You cannot control your biology. But you can control how you communicate your needs, set your boundaries, and educate the people in your life.

This is not easy. It requires you to be vulnerable, brave, and sometimes uncomfortably direct. But building a team of allies who understand your condition and know how to support you is one of the most powerful things you can do to improve your quality of life. An understanding friend is as valuable as a good rescue medication. A partner who knows how to create a calm space is as critical as a blackout curtain.

Do this before the week is out. Not someday. This week.

Pick one person.

Just one. Your partner, your best friend, your mom, your boss. The person whose support would make the biggest difference. Schedule a time to have "The Talk"---on a good day, when you're feeling strong. Use the scripts in this chapter. Forward them the FAQ. Share the Quick Guide Card that matches their role. Open the lines of communication before the next crisis hits.

Building your support crew is just as important as stocking your medicine cabinet. It's the infrastructure that will hold you up when you feel like you're about to collapse.

You've now learned how to engineer your environment and advocate for yourself in your personal life. But what about the biggest, most intimidating system of all? In the next section, PART V: ADVOCATE, we're going to zoom out. It's time to learn how to hack the beast that is the healthcare and insurance system.

Chapter 11: Hacking the Healthcare System

Navigating Doctors & Insurance

Welcome to Part V. You've learned to understand, anticipate, act, and engineer your world. Now for the final bosses.

But now, you face the final bosses: the Doctor and the Insurance Company.

These are not villains to be vanquished. They are complex, bureaucratic systems with their own languages and motivations. Navigating them—the 15-minute appointment slots, the arcane billing codes, the phone trees designed by sadists—can feel more exhausting than a three-day migraine hangover.

This chapter is your cheat code. It's your hacking manual. We are going to transform you from a patient into a project manager, from a supplicant into a CEO. You are the leader of "Project: My Health," and your doctor is a highly specialized, brilliant, but incredibly busy consultant. The insurance company is your board of investors---skeptical, budget-conscious, and in need of a very convincing business case.

Your mission, should you choose to accept it, is to become the most prepared, most articulate, most effective expert in the room. Especially when that room has a doctor in it.

📖 Ken's Corner: Five Years, Eight Doctors, and One Lesson Nobody Teaches You

You've already heard my story — nearly five years, eight doctors, a trip to Mayo Clinic, and a structural diagnosis that was hiding in my own imaging the whole time (see the Introduction if you need the full version). The point of retelling it here isn't the drama. It's the lesson: the healthcare system is not designed to see you whole. It sees you in specialty-sized slices. Your neurologist sees the neurology. Your orthopedic surgeon sees the spine. Nobody is automatically assigned to hold the full picture of your symptoms, your imaging, your treatment history, and your lived experience. That job is yours. And these tools will help you do it.

How to "Speak Doctor": A Crash Course in Clinical Communication

The average doctor's appointment lasts about 15 minutes. In that time, your doctor has to listen, diagnose, plan, and document. It's an impossible task.

Patients who show up saying "my head hurts a lot" walk away with vague solutions. Patients who show up with data get results.

You are not there to "chat." You are there to deliver an executive briefing. Here's how.

Preparation is 90% of the Battle

You would never walk into a critical business meeting unprepared. Don't do it with your health. The work you do before your appointment is what will determine its success. This is where your Migraine Dashboard (from Chapter 5) earns its keep. You need to distill all that rich data into a single, powerful document.

TOOL: The Printable Doctor Visit Planner

This isn't just a list of questions; it's your entire meeting agenda on a single page. It's the document you will physically hand to your doctor or their nurse at the beginning of your appointment. It shows you are prepared, organized, and respectful of their time. It immediately elevates you from "just another patient" to a partner in your own care. In the Field Manual at the end of this book, you'll find a full-page, fillable version of this to print out.

The Ultimate Doctor Visit Planner

Patient Name: ______________ Date of Visit: _______________

1. The Headline (My Goal for Today's Visit): (In one sentence, what is the #1 thing you need to accomplish?)

- Example: "To discuss why my current rescue medication, Sumatriptan, is no longer effective and to explore options like CGRP inhibitors."

2. The Vital Stats (The Last 30 Days): (This is your data snapshot)

- Number of Migraine Attack Days: ____
- Average Pain Intensity (1-10 Scale): ____
- Top 3 Suspected Triggers This Month: 1. ________ 2. ________ 3. ________
- My Most Debilitating Symptoms Are: ____________________

3. Treatment History & Effectiveness: (What have you tried and how did it go?)

Current Rescue Med: [e.g., Sumatriptan 100mg]

Effectiveness: Works ____% of the time.

Side Effects: [e.g., Chest tightness, fatigue]

Current Preventive Med: [e.g., Propranolol 80mg]

Effectiveness: [e.g., Reduced attack days from 15 to 12]

Side Effects: [e.g., Dizziness, low energy]

Supplements/Other: [e.g., Magnesium Glycinate 400mg, effective for sleep]

4. My Top 3 Questions (In Order of Importance): (Write them down so you don't forget!)

- 1.
- 2.
- 3.

5. My Desired Outcome / Next Steps: (What do you hope to leave with?)

- Example: "A prescription for a new preventive, a referral to a physical therapist for my neck pain, and a plan for my next follow-up."

Speaking the Language: Data, Assertiveness, and "The Loop"

With your Planner in hand, you are ready for the visit itself.

- Lead the Conversation: The moment the doctor walks in and asks, "So, what brings you in today?" is your moment. Don't meander. Hand them your Planner and say:

"Thanks for seeing me. I've prepared a one-page summary to make the best use of our time. The main goal for today is to discuss..." You have just taken control of the meeting and framed yourself as an organized, serious partner.

Speak in Numbers: Doctors think in data. Replace vague, emotional language with cold, hard facts from your diary.

Instead of: "I feel like I'm getting migraines all the time now."

Say: "My migraine frequency has increased from 8 days a month to 14 days a month over the last quarter."

Instead of: "My medication doesn't really work that well."

Say: "According to my log, my sumatriptan only reduces my pain by 50% or more in 3 out of 10 attacks."

- Be Assertive, Not Aggressive: There is a huge difference. Aggression is demanding and puts the doctor on the defensive. Assertiveness is confidently and calmly stating your experience, needs, and boundaries.

Aggressive: "You have to give me something better! This stuff you prescribed is useless."

- Assertive: "The current treatment isn't meeting my goals for quality of life. The side effects are significant, and it's only providing minimal relief. I'd like to talk about the next step in my treatment plan, such as [mention a therapy you've researched, e.g., 'a CGRP inhibitor']."
- Close the Loop: At the end of the appointment, before you walk out the door, summarize the plan back to the doctor. This ensures you both have the same understanding and clarifies any confusion.

"Okay, just to make sure I have this right: the plan is for me to start taking Topiramate at 25mg, increase the dose next week, continue tracking my symptoms, and we'll follow up in six weeks. Is that correct?"

This simple act can prevent months of misunderstanding and incorrect treatment.

The Secret Language: Your ICD-10 Code Cheat Sheet

What's an ICD-10 code? It's the alphanumeric code that doctors use to classify your diagnosis for billing and medical records. It's part of the secret language of the healthcare system. Why should you care? Because having the correct and most specific code on your chart is crucial for getting insurance to approve the treatments you need.

If your chart just says "Headache," you're going to have a hard time getting Botox for Chronic Migraine approved. You need to ensure your doctor is using the code that accurately reflects your condition.

TOOL: The Migraine Warrior's ICD-10 Cheat Sheet

You don't need to be a medical coder, but knowing these can help you have an informed conversation with your doctor's billing office or check your own records.

G43.909 - Migraine, unspecified, not intractable, without status migrainosus: The generic, basic code for migraine.

G43.009 - Migraine with aura, not intractable, without status migrainosus: For the "Drama Queens."

G43.109 - Migraine without aura, not intractable, without status migrainosus: For the "Silent Ninjas."

- G43.709 - Chronic migraine without aura, not intractable, without status migrainosus: THIS IS A KEY ONE. If you have 15 or more headache days a month, this diagnosis is often required for treatments like Botox.

G44.209 - Tension-type headache, unspecified, not intractable: The code for the "annoying intern."

G50.0 - Trigeminal neuralgia: The code for the "face's fury."

M54.2 - Cervicalgia: The code for neck pain, often used alongside migraine when there is a neck component.

You can politely ask your doctor, "For my records, could you confirm the specific diagnosis code you're using? I want to make sure it accurately reflects the frequency and nature of my attacks for my insurance."

The Insurance Gauntlet: A Bureaucratic Survival Guide

You've done it. You've prepared your data, you've mastered the art of "speaking doctor," and you and your physician have decided on a new, promising, and probably very expensive treatment plan. You feel a glimmer of hope.

And then you get a notification from your pharmacy: "Prior Authorization Required."

Welcome to the gauntlet. This is the part of the journey where your medical needs meet the cold, hard reality of corporate finance. The insurance system is a bureaucratic beast, a labyrinth of policies, exclusions, and phone trees designed to wear you down. But here's the secret: it's just a game. A very annoying, high-stakes game, but a game nonetheless. And like any game, it has rules you can learn and strategies you can use to win.

Think of yourself as a warrior entering a dungeon. The dungeon is filled with traps (denials), puzzles (paperwork), and a final boss (the appeals committee). Your mission is to get the treasure (the treatment you need) without losing your sanity.

The Gatekeeper: Understanding Prior Authorization

A Prior Authorization (PA) is exactly what it sounds like. Before your insurance company agrees to pay for a specific, often newer or more expensive medication or procedure, they require your doctor to get prior approval. They want your doctor to submit a detailed business case proving why you, specifically, need this fancy treatment instead of the cheaper ones they'd rather you use.

- The "Step Therapy" Trap: The most common reason for a PA is a process called "step therapy" or "fail first." Your insurance company has a list of preferred, older, and (most importantly) cheaper drugs. They will require you to try and "fail" on one or two of these drugs before they will even consider approving the newer, more effective one your doctor actually prescribed.

- Why this is infuriating: You and your doctor know that a beta-blocker might not be right for you, but you may have to spend three miserable months on it just to get the denial on paper. This is a frustrating reality, but it's a hoop you often have to jump through.

How to Win the PA Game:

- Be Your Doctor's Admin Assistant: The PA process is a massive administrative burden on your doctor's office. You can be an invaluable part of the team. Make sure they have a crystal-clear, detailed history of every single medication you have tried and why it failed. Did it not work? Did it give you unbearable side effects? Document it all in your diary. This data is the evidence your doctor needs to prove you've "failed" the required steps.
- Become a Polite Nuisance: This is a delicate art. You need to follow up---with your doctor's office and the insurance company---persistently. A weekly, polite phone call ("Hi, just checking on the status of my prior authorization for [Medication Name]") keeps your case from falling through the cracks. Remember, the squeaky wheel gets the grease, but a rude wheel gets its case file "accidentally" put at the bottom of the pile.

The Final Boss: The Appeal Process

So, they denied your prior authorization. You got the letter in the mail, filled with cold, corporate jargon. Your first instinct is probably a combination of rage and despair. Allow yourself a moment to feel that. Scream into a pillow if you must.

Now, take a deep breath and put on your battle armor. A denial is not the end. It is simply the beginning of the appeals process.

- Level 1: The Internal Appeal: Your first step is to file an appeal directly with the insurance company. This is usually reviewed by a different medical director within the same company. Your doctor's office will handle the submission, but your job is to help them build an ironclad case. This includes:
- A Letter of Medical Necessity from Your Doctor: This is the core of your appeal. Your doctor will outline your medical history, the treatments you've failed, and the clinical rationale for why the requested treatment is medically necessary for you.

- Your Personal Impact Statement: This is your secret weapon. You will write a one-page letter explaining, in your own words, how migraines have impacted your life. Don't just talk about pain. Talk about the days of work you've missed. The school events you couldn't attend. The toll it's taken on your family and your mental health. Make them see the human cost. An adjuster can deny a claim number, but it's much harder to deny a compelling human story.
- All The Data: Include summary reports from your migraine app. Include a printed log of your attacks. Include everything. Drown them in evidence of your suffering and your diligent attempts to get better.
- Level 2: The External Review: If the internal appeal is denied (which can happen), you can request an external review. This is where your case is sent to an independent, third-party organization of doctors who have no affiliation with your insurance company. They will review the case impartially. Your chances of winning at this stage are often much higher, especially if your case is well-documented.

The key to all of this is documentation and persistence. It's a war of attrition. The insurance company is betting you'll get tired and give up. Don't.

TOOL: The Sample Prior Authorization / Appeal Letter

Use this template as a starting point. You and your doctor can adapt it to fit your specific situation. This letter is designed to be clear, professional, and impossible to ignore.

[Your Doctor's Letterhead]

[Date]

[Insurance Company's Name] [Prior Authorization/Appeals Department] [Address]

RE: Letter of Medical Necessity for [Patient Name] Patient Name: [Your Full Name] Patient DOB: [Your Date of Birth] Policy/ID Number: [Your Insurance ID Number] Requested Treatment: [e.g., Emgality (galcanezumab) 120 mg/mL injection]

To Whom It May Concern:

I am writing on behalf of my patient, [Your Name], to request prior authorization for [Medication Name] for the treatment of their diagnosed Chronic Migraine (ICD-10: G43.709). This treatment is medically necessary and is the most appropriate course of action due to the severity of the patient's condition and their documented failure to respond to multiple other therapies.

Patient History & Diagnosis: [Your Name] is a [Your Age]-year-old patient who has suffered from debilitating migraines for [Number] years. They currently experience an average of [Number, e.g., 18] migraine days per month, with an average pain intensity of 8/10. These attacks are accompanied by severe nausea, photophobia, and phonophobia, significantly impacting their ability to work, care for their family, and engage in daily life activities. (Optional: "Please see attached patient impact statement for further detail.")

History of Failed Therapies (Step Therapy Documentation): In accordance with your step therapy policy, the patient has trialed and failed the following preventive medications due to lack of efficacy and/or intolerable side effects:

- [Medication 1, e.g., Propranolol]: Dosed up to [Dose, e.g., 120mg/day]. Tripled for [Duration, e.g., 4 months] from [Start Date] to [End Date]. Result: No significant reduction in migraine frequency. Side Effects: [e.g., Severe fatigue, dizziness].
- [Medication 2, e.g., Topiramate]: Dosed up to [Dose, e.g., 100mg/day]. Tripled for [Duration, e.g., 3 months] from [Start Date] to [End Date]. Result: Patient was unable to tolerate due to significant cognitive side effects ("brain fog") that interfered with their employment.

[Medication 3, e.g., Amitriptyline]: [Provide similar details].

(Please see attached medical records and migraine diary logs for detailed documentation of these treatment failures.)

Clinical Rationale for [Requested Medication]: Given the patient's failure to respond to or tolerate multiple classes of older preventive medications, a CGRP monoclonal antibody is the clear and evidence-based next step. [Medication Name] is a targeted therapy specifically designed for migraine prevention and has been shown in numerous clinical trials to be highly effective and well-tolerated in patients like [Your Name]. Continuing to deny access to this treatment will only result in further suffering, disability, and increased healthcare utilization (e.g., emergency room visits).

This treatment is not experimental; it is the standard of care for refractory chronic migraine. I have attached relevant peer-reviewed studies supporting its use in this patient population.

Please approve this request for [Medication Name] for [Your Name] as expeditiously as possible. If you require any further information, please do not hesitate to contact my office at [Doctor's Phone Number].

Sincerely,

[Doctor's Signature]

[Doctor's Printed Name, M.D./D.O.] [Doctor's NPI Number]

TOOL: A Letter to Your Medical Team

The following is a template adapted from my own journey. It's designed for patients who have been in the system a long time, suspect a structural or atypical component to their headache disorder, and want to communicate that clearly and respectfully without being dismissed. Customize it. Use the parts that fit your story. Leave the parts that don't.

[Date]

Dear [Doctor's Name],

Thank you for seeing me. I want to make the best use of our time together, and I want to be honest with you about where I am in this process.

I have been managing significant head pain and associated neurological symptoms for approximately [X] years. During that time, I have been evaluated and treated by [number] providers, including [brief list, e.g., two neurologists, a pain specialist, and a team at a major academic medical center]. I have trialed [list key medications], with limited or partial benefit. I am grateful for everything those providers offered. I am also still in pain.

I am not writing this to challenge any prior diagnosis or to suggest that previous care was inadequate. I am writing this because I believe there may be aspects of my symptom picture that haven't yet been fully integrated, and I would like your help looking at the whole picture.

The symptoms I am most concerned about, which I don't believe fit the standard migraine profile cleanly:

- [List your specific atypical symptoms -- e.g., facial or scalp numbness, symptoms that worsen predictably with specific physical activities or positions, arm weakness, symptoms that respond partially but incompletely to migraine-specific treatments]

The imaging findings I would like to discuss:

- [Reference specific findings from existing imaging -- e.g., "My [year] MRI showed [finding]. My [year] CT showed [finding]. I would like to understand whether these findings may be contributing to my symptoms."]

What I am asking for:

I am not asking you to agree with any particular hypothesis. I am asking for a conversation about whether the structural findings in my imaging are clinically relevant to my symptom picture, and whether referral to [e.g., a spine specialist, interventional pain provider, or neurosurgeon] for further evaluation might be appropriate.

I am a motivated, engaged patient. I track my symptoms, I take my medications as prescribed, and I follow through on recommendations. I am asking you to be a partner in finding an answer, not just a manager of ongoing symptoms.

Thank you for your time and for reading this. I look forward to talking with you.

Sincerely,

[Your Name]

[Contact Information]

[List of attached documents, e.g., recent migraine diary summary, imaging reports, prior treatment records]

Conclusion: You Are the CEO

Let's be real: navigating the healthcare system can feel like a full-time job you never applied for and certainly don't get paid for. It's a world of red tape, confusing terminology, and soul-crushing bureaucracy.

You now have the tools to lead your own healthcare. You are the CEO of "Project: My Health." Data is your leverage, clear communication is your strategy, and persistence is your superpower. You know how to walk into a doctor's office not as a list of symptoms, but as a prepared partner. You know how to look at an insurance denial not as a verdict, but as an invitation to appeal.

And now you know something else too: the system is fragmented by design. Specialists see slices. You see the whole. Your job is to hold the full picture of your own experience, carry it into every room, and find the providers who are willing to sit with you and look at it together.

That is what it means to advocate. It's not easy, but it is the path to getting the care you deserve.

Go get a folder or a binder. Label it "My Doctor Go-Bag."

Inside, I want you to put three things, right now.

- Print out the Doctor Visit Planner from the Field Manual at the end of this book and fill it out as best you can for your next appointment, even if it's months away.

On a separate piece of paper, write down the top three questions you have about your current treatment plan.

- Print out a one-month summary report from your migraine tracking app, or make a copy of your last month's paper diary entries.

That's it. You have now created your official summit portfolio. The next time you have an appointment, you won't just be showing up. You'll be arriving prepared, armed with data, and ready to lead.

You have now learned how to advocate for yourself within the system. But what happens when your symptoms don't fit the classic migraine mold? In the next chapter, we're going to meet the impostors and co-conspirators---the comorbidities and copycats that can make diagnosis so challenging.

Chapter 12: The Usual Suspects

Comorbidities & Copycats

You're armed with data and you know how to use it. But what happens when the clues don't add up? When your "migraine" doesn't play by the rules, or brings a whole gang of other symptoms along for the ride?

Welcome to the police lineup of neurology. This is where we investigate the "usual suspects"---the other medical conditions that love to hang out with migraine, and the impostors that try to wear its face.

Think of your migraine as the charismatic, headline-grabbing crime boss. For some people, it acts alone. But for many of us, it's the head of a whole criminal syndicate. It has co-conspirators, lookalikes, and copycats. Your job as the lead detective on your own case is to figure out if you're dealing with a lone wolf or an entire mob.

Why? Because if you're only treating the crime boss, you'll never get peace. You have to understand the whole network. This chapter is your informant. It's the insider guide to the complex web of comorbidities (the co-conspirators) and differential diagnoses (the copycats) that can make getting the right treatment feel like a medical mystery novel. This is advanced-level self-advocacy. Let's identify the crew.

The Frequent Co-Conspirators: When Migraine Doesn't Travel Alone

First, a term: comorbidity. It's when two or more conditions shack up in the same body more often than random chance explains. They share underlying mechanisms—a dysfunctional autonomic nervous system, chronic inflammation, or a brain that's wound too tight (central sensitization).

Recognizing a potential co-conspirator is a game-changer. It can explain a whole constellation of weird symptoms you thought were unrelated and open up entirely new avenues for treatment.

1. POTS (Postural Orthostatic Tachycardia Syndrome)

- What It Is, Snarky Edition: POTS is what happens when your body's gravity sensor is broken. Standing up, for you, is an extreme sport. Your autonomic nervous system---the body's automatic control panel for things like heart rate and blood pressure---forgets what to do when you go from sitting to standing. Your blood vessels don't constrict properly, so blood pools in your lower body, and your heart starts beating like a drum solo trying to get blood back up to your brain.
- The Link to Migraine: Both are disorders of the autonomic nervous system (dysautonomia). The poor blood flow to the brain in POTS can be a major migraine trigger. Many people with POTS experience chronic daily headaches that feel like migraines.

Symptoms to Watch For:

- A rapid increase in heart rate upon standing (the defining feature).
- Dizziness, lightheadedness, or even fainting when you stand up.
- Chronic fatigue, brain fog, and exercise intolerance.
- Feeling drastically better when you lie down.

2. Fibromyalgia

- What It Is, Snarky Edition: Fibromyalgia is when your body's volume knob for pain is permanently stuck at 11. It's a condition of widespread, chronic pain, accompanied by fatigue and cognitive issues. It's like your entire nervous system is one big, oversensitive, bruised nerve.
- The Link to Migraine: The connection is central sensitization. In both fibromyalgia and chronic migraine, the brain and spinal cord become incredibly efficient at amplifying pain signals. Normal stimuli that shouldn't hurt, like a light touch or moderate exercise, are interpreted as painful. Your nervous systems are essentially professional drama queens.

Symptoms to Watch For:

- Widespread, dull, aching pain that lasts for months.
- Specific tender points on the body.
- Profound fatigue that isn't relieved by sleep.

- "Fibro fog"---difficulty with memory and concentration.

3. Anxiety & Depression

- What They Are, Snarky Edition: The unwelcome mental roommates that often come with the chronic illness territory. Anxiety is the voice that whispers, "What if it happens again?" Depression is the heavy blanket that tells you, "What's the point of even trying?"
- The Link to Migraine: This is a two-way street of misery. Living with chronic, unpredictable pain is inherently anxiety-inducing and depressing. On a biological level, migraines and mood disorders share the same neurotransmitter pathways. Serotonin and norepinephrine, which regulate mood, are also critical for regulating pain. When they're out of whack, you get a double whammy of both physical and emotional pain.

Symptoms to Watch For:

Anxiety: Constant worry, restlessness, panic attacks, avoiding situations for fear of a trigger.

- Depression: Persistent low mood, loss of interest in things you once enjoyed, changes in sleep or appetite, feelings of hopelessness.

4. ADHD (Attention-Deficit/Hyperactivity Disorder)

- What It Is, Snarky Edition: The "my brain has too many tabs open" disorder. It's a neurodevelopmental condition characterized by issues with executive function---things like focus, organization, emotional regulation, and impulse control.
- The Link to Migraine: The connection is still being researched, but it's strong. Both conditions involve dysregulation of neurotransmitters, particularly dopamine. There's also a theory that the sensory hypersensitivity common in ADHD (being overwhelmed by sounds, lights, and textures) overlaps significantly with the photophobia and phonophobia of migraine, suggesting a shared issue with sensory processing.

Symptoms to Watch For:

- Difficulty sustaining attention, especially on boring tasks.
- Procrastination and trouble with time management.

- Impulsivity or restlessness.
- Being easily overwhelmed in busy environments.

5. Neck Problems & The Neuralgias

- What They Are, Snarky Edition: This is when your head isn't the problem; it's the scaffolding that holds it up. Your neck, with its complex web of muscles and nerves, can become a primary source of pain that your brain interprets as a migraine. Occipital and Trigeminal Neuralgia are the lead villains here.
- The Link to Migraine: Structural issues in the neck (cervicogenic problems) or irritated nerves (neuralgias) can send a constant barrage of pain signals to the trigeminal nucleus in your brainstem. This is the same command center that processes migraine pain. When this area gets overwhelmed with signals from your neck, it can kick off a true migraine attack. It's a classic case of mistaken identity and overreaction. We'll dive deeper into these impostors in a moment.

The Impostors: Unmasking the Migraine Lookalikes

Sometimes, what you think is a migraine is actually a completely different condition wearing a very convincing costume. Getting the right diagnosis here is everything, because the treatments are often entirely different. This is where you, the detective, need to pay close attention to the specific nature of the clues.

1. Occipital & Trigeminal Neuralgia (The Nerve Impostors)

As we mentioned, these are frequent co-conspirators, but they are also master impostors.

Occipital Neuralgia (ON): This is pain from the occipital nerves being squeezed or irritated at the back of your neck.

- The Telltale Sign: The pain quality. It is NOT a deep throb. It is a sharp, zapping, shooting, electric-shock pain that radiates from the base of your skull up the back of your head. The scalp itself is often exquisitely tender to the touch.

Trigeminal Neuralgia (TN): This is pain from the trigeminal nerve itself, usually due to a blood vessel compressing it.

- The Telltale Sign: The triggers. The pain is an excruciating, electric stab in the FACE (not the head) brought on by the lightest touch---a breeze, brushing your teeth, a kiss.

2. TMJ Disorder (The Mechanical Impostor)

- What It Is: A disorder of your temporomandibular joint---your jaw joint. It can be caused by teeth grinding (bruxism), jaw clenching, or misalignment.
- How it Mimics Migraine: The major muscles involved in chewing (like the temporalis muscle) span across your temples. When these muscles are overworked and inflamed from TMJ issues, they can create a headache that feels remarkably like a one-sided, temporal migraine.
- The Telltale Sign: Your headache is accompanied by jaw-specific symptoms: a clicking or popping sound when you open your mouth, jaw pain or stiffness (especially in the morning), or pain when chewing.

3. IIH - Idiopathic Intracranial Hypertension (The Pressure Impostor)

- What It Is: A condition where the pressure inside your skull is too high for no obvious reason (that's the "idiopathic" part). It's sometimes called pseudotumor cerebri because it mimics the symptoms of a brain tumor without the actual tumor.
- How it Mimics Migraine: The primary symptom is a severe, often daily, headache. The pain is often described as pulsating and can be worsened by activity. Sound familiar?

The Telltale Signs:

- Vision Changes: This is the key differentiator. The high pressure pushes on your optic nerves, which can cause transient visual obscurations (your vision briefly dimming or going out, especially when you bend over), double vision, and, in serious cases, permanent vision loss. An eye doctor can see swelling of the optic nerve (papilledema) during an exam.

Pulsatile Tinnitus: A "whooshing" sound in your ears that is in time with your heartbeat.

The Symptom Cluster Matrix: Your Lineup of Suspects

Use this matrix to compare your constellation of symptoms against the classic profiles. If a column other than "Classic Migraine" starts to feel uncomfortably familiar, it's a major clue that you need to have a deeper conversation with your doctor.

TOOL: The Symptom Cluster Matrix

🕮 Ken's Corner: When Migraine Is the Wrong Label

I want to tell you about the day I stopped having migraines. Not because they went away. Because I finally understood what I actually had. For years, the working diagnosis was migraine — and the evidence for it was reasonable. What nobody was asking was why the standard treatments kept only getting me halfway there. My symptom picture, in retrospect, should have been pointing somewhere structural all along. The features that didn't fit classic migraine — the positional triggers, the facial numbness, the load-dependent pain — were breadcrumbs leading to the cervical spine. The distinction matters because the treatment is different. You cannot fully resolve a structurally-driven pain pattern with medications designed for a neurochemically-driven one. If any of this resonates, ask the question. Bring your imaging. Find someone willing to look at the scaffolding, not just the alarm it's setting off.

When to Push for More: Advocacy in Action

You've reviewed the lineup. You've studied the Symptom Cluster Matrix. And maybe, just maybe, a little lightbulb has gone off in your foggy brain. Maybe you've realized that your "migraine" has some unusual features that don't quite fit the classic profile.

This is a critical moment. It's the point in the investigation where a good detective says, "We need to bring in another expert." In your case, this means knowing when to push your doctor for a referral to a different specialist or for specific diagnostic imaging.

This isn't about questioning your doctor's expertise; it's about being a proactive partner in your own care. You are the one living in your body 24/7. You are the world's leading expert on your own symptoms. If your gut tells you there's more to the story, it's time to listen.

Here are the clear signs that it's time to advocate for a deeper look.

When to Push for a Specialist Referral

Your primary care doctor or even your general neurologist is a fantastic starting point, but some conditions require a highly specialized eye. You should consider asking for a referral if:

- Your primary symptom is dizziness, not pain. If the spinning, vertigo, and disequilibrium are the main event and the headache is just a minor guest star (or doesn't show up at all), you need to ask for a referral to a Vestibular Specialist. This could be a neurologist with extra training in dizziness, an otolaryngologist (ENT), or a specialized physical therapist. They have the tools to diagnose and treat conditions like Vestibular Migraine or other inner-ear issues.
- You feel faint, and your heart races every time you stand up. If the description of POTS felt uncomfortably familiar, it's time to see a Cardiologist or a Neurologist specializing in Dysautonomia. They can perform a tilt table test to get a definitive diagnosis and explore treatments like beta-blockers, hydration protocols, and compression garments that can drastically improve your quality of life (and potentially reduce your migraine load).
- You have widespread body pain, profound fatigue, and brain fog. If you checked off every box for Fibromyalgia, a referral to a Rheumatologist is in order. They specialize in musculoskeletal and autoimmune conditions and can help differentiate fibro from other things like lupus or rheumatoid arthritis, creating a treatment plan that addresses both the body pain and the migraines.
- Your pain is a distinct, electric ZAP that starts in your neck. If the Occipital Neuralgia description made you shout "THAT'S IT!" at this book, you need to see a Pain Management Specialist or a Neurologist who specializes in nerve blocks and interventional procedures. Standard migraine medications often fail for pure ON. You need someone who can go after the irritated nerve itself with tools like nerve blocks or ablations.
- Your headache is always accompanied by jaw pain, clicking, or locking. If the TMJ profile fits you to a T, you need to see a specialist, but it might not be an M.D. Ask your dentist

for a referral to a TMJ Specialist or an Oral and Maxillofacial Surgeon. They can assess your bite and jaw mechanics and recommend treatments like custom mouthguards or physical therapy.

- Your headache gets dramatically worse when you lie down and you have vision changes. If the IIH description gave you pause, you need to see a Neuro-ophthalmologist. This is a super-specialist who is both a neurologist and an eye doctor. They are the ultimate experts in conditions that link the brain and the eyes and are best equipped to diagnose and manage IIH to protect your vision.

ACTION BOX: When to Ask for an MRI (A Guide for Your Doctor Conversation)

Let's be crystal clear: you should not demand an MRI just because your head hurts. It's not a magic migraine-finding machine. In fact, for a standard migraine, an MRI will look completely normal. Its purpose is not to diagnose migraine; its purpose is to rule out other scary things. This checklist is to help you identify red flags that warrant a serious conversation with your doctor about whether imaging is medically necessary.

Consider asking your doctor about an MRI if your headache is...

- [ ] The "Thunderclap": Came on suddenly and explosively, reaching maximum, unbearable intensity in under 60 seconds. This is a medical emergency to rule out a brain bleed.
- [ ] Accompanied by New, Alarming Neurological Signs: You're experiencing symptoms you've never had before that aren't part of a typical aura, such as a seizure, persistent weakness on one side of your body, personality changes, or profound confusion.
- [ ] A Brand New Headache After Age 50: If you've never had migraines and suddenly develop a new, severe type of headache after the age of 50, imaging is often recommended to rule out other causes.
- [ ] Changing with Position: The pain gets dramatically worse or better when you lie down versus when you stand up. This can be a sign of a pressure issue, like IIH or a CSF leak.

- [ ] Showing a Significant, Unexplained Pattern Change: You've had migraines for years, but this is different. The location, quality, or severity has fundamentally changed, and it's getting progressively worse over weeks or months.
- [ ] Accompanied by Systemic Symptoms: The headache comes with other red flags like a high fever, a stiff neck, or an unexplained rash, which could signal an infection like meningitis.

Disclaimer: This is a tool for patient education and advocacy, not a diagnostic manual. The decision to order an MRI rests solely with your qualified medical provider based on a full clinical evaluation.

Chapter Twelve Conclusion: You Are the Lead Investigator

We've just journeyed through the criminal underworld of neurology, unmasking the accomplices and impostors that complicate the migraine case. It can feel overwhelming to realize that your body might be hosting not just one, but an entire syndicate of dysfunctional conditions.

But I want you to reframe that feeling. This is not overwhelming; this is empowering.

You are no longer operating on the single, simple theory that "it's just a migraine." You are now a lead investigator with a whole new set of leads to follow. You understand that the dizziness might be POTS, that the neck pain might be ON, that the vision changes might be IIH. You have a map, and you have a list of suspects.

Your pain and your constellation of weird symptoms are not random. They are clues. And you, the person living with them every single day, are the one best equipped to notice them. Your detailed observations are more valuable than any single lab test or scan.

One last thing before you move on.

Go back and look at the Symptom Cluster Matrix one more time. Read through it slowly. Is there a box, a symptom, a single phrase that made you pause and think, "Huh. That sounds... familiar"?

If the answer is yes, I want you to grab your Doctor Visit Planner from the last chapter. In the section titled "My Top 3 Questions," I want you to write this down:

"My symptoms also include [symptom you circled]. Based on my research, I'm wondering if we should explore the possibility of [condition from the matrix]? What are your thoughts?"

That's it. That's the entire assignment. By writing down that one question, you are taking a monumental step. You are moving beyond simply reporting your symptoms and into the realm of collaborative diagnosis. You are bringing your expertise---the lived experience of your own body---to the table as a valid and crucial piece of evidence.

You're not just a patient anymore. You're the lead investigator on your own case. Now go solve it.

With your advocacy skills sharpened, there's only one place left to look: forward. In our final chapter, we'll explore the cutting edge of research, the brilliant innovations on the horizon, and the very real reason we all have to be hopeful for the future of migraine care.

Chapter 13: The Hope Horizon

Research, Trials & the Future

We've been through it all, haven't we? We've stared into the abyss of our own neurology, mapped the battlefields, built our arsenals, and learned to advocate for ourselves in a world that often just doesn't get it. It's a hard-fought, grinding, day-in-day-out war.

It's easy to get lost in that trench warfare. It's easy to believe that this---the constant vigilance, the pain, the fatigue---is all there is.

This chapter is your order to stop, put down your weapon for a moment, and lift your head. It's time to look at the horizon. Because for the first time in the history of this ancient, miserable disease, the future is not just a vague, distant hope. It is bright. It is tangible. And it is coming fast.

For centuries, migraine treatment was a clumsy affair of borrowed drugs and blind guesses. We were fighting a neurological electrical fire with a bucket of water and a prayer. Not anymore. We are now living in the single most exciting era of migraine research the world has ever known. The science has finally caught up to our suffering, and the brilliant minds in labs around the globe are building us better weapons.

This chapter is your sneak peek into their workshops. It's a snapshot of the sci-fi-level technology and biology that is no longer decades away, but is in pipelines right now. This isn't about "miracle cures." This is about real, evidence-based progress. This is your dose of optimism, backed by science. So let's take a look at the future, shall we?

📖 Ken's Corner: The Night I Got My Answer from a Machine

I want to tell you about a Tuesday night that changed my life. It wasn't a doctor's appointment. It wasn't a breakthrough drug or a new specialist. It was me, alone at my computer at some ridiculous hour, finally doing something I'd been putting off for months: uploading my old MRI & CT imaging files to an AI.

I had been in pain for nearly five years. I had seen eight doctors. I had four rounds of occipital nerve blocks, each helping a little, each wearing off. I had been to Mayo Clinic. I had a drawer full of medications that had worked partially, or not at all, or worked and then stopped. I had a diagnosis -- migraine -- that fit the surface symptoms but never explained the full picture. The facial numbness. The arm weakness. The pain that spiked when I bent over to look under my car or held my arms overhead. The scalp tenderness so specific I could point to the exact spot.

I was exhausted in the way that only people who have been chronically ill for years can understand. Not just physically but mentally. Suicidal thoughts briefly flying through my mind's eye wondering if ending it all would finally get rid of this daily nagging non-stop pain. Worrying that I would take this pain with me to the next realm as punishment. You know, the particular exhaustion of having been believed but not solved. Of having worked the system correctly -- tracking, documenting, advocating -- and still finding yourself in the same dark room, ice pack or heating pad on your neck, wondering if this is just who you are now.

That Tuesday, I uploaded my MRI and CT reports I'd accumulated over the years to an AI chat interface. Old scans. Some from years before. The ones that had been read, filed, and never mentioned again in any appointment. I asked it to tell me what it saw.

What came back stopped me cold.

The AI walked me through the findings systematically. Multilevel cervical spondylosis with disc-osteophyte complexes at C2-3, C3-4, and C5-6. C2-4 facet arthrosis. Posterior bone spurs at those same levels. And then the one that made everything click into place: severe right-sided foraminal stenosis at C5-C6 -- a narrowing significant enough to compress the nerve root that runs through it.

I sat there reading the summary and felt something shift in my chest. Not panic. Recognition. I cried from joy, finally a potential solution to all of this.

I printed the conversation. I brought it to a surgeon.

He reviewed the old imaging himself, he immediately ordered new imaging, both MRI and CT scans. I saw him a week later and he confirmed the AI's suspicion and his. He agreed the cervical findings were significant and potentially symptomatic. He ordered diagnostic injections at the C2-C6 levels, in two separate sessions a month apart -- not to treat, but to diagnose: if anesthetizing those facet joints reduced the pain, that was our answer. If it didn't, we kept looking.

The injection was one of the stranger experiences of my life. Within a few days, after the initial vestibular fallout from the procedure settled, something happened that I hadn't felt in years. The background noise went quiet.

Not silent. Not cured. But the low, constant undertone of pain that I had stopped noticing because it had become the baseline -- it dimmed. I remembered what it felt like to not be bracing. I had a few days that felt almost like being my old self. I cried hard, I could get my old life back, I finally for once in 5 years had hope!

Then I pushed my luck with some physical work around the house and the cervical loading flared everything back up, which was, perversely, more confirmation. The spine was the source. We had a diagnosis within a diagnosis. ACDF or ADR surgery was being discussed.

I am not on the other side of this story yet. I'm in it. The surgery hasn't happened. The full resolution is still ahead of me. I'm telling you this now, before that chapter is written, because I want you to understand something important.

The turning point in my five-year journey was not a doctor. It was a tool. An AI reading imaging reports that had been sitting in my chart, unconnected, for years.

I am not saying this to diminish the doctors who helped me along the way. Several of them were excellent within the scope of their specialty. I am saying this because we are living in a moment where the technology available to patients outside the clinical encounter has become genuinely, meaningfully diagnostic. Not a replacement for medical care. Not a substitute for a surgeon who can look at a scan and a patient together and make a judgment call. But a powerful bridge.

If you have years of imaging sitting in your portal, unexamined after the initial read -- upload it. Ask questions. The AI doesn't have a 15-minute appointment slot. It doesn't have a differential diagnosis it's already committed to. It will look at everything you give it and tell you what it sees.

I can't promise you'll find what I found. Your answer may be purely neurochemical. Your migraine may be exactly the diagnosis it appears to be, and the path forward may be through the treatments in Chapter 7 rather than an operating room. That's okay. That's a valid and treatable story.

But if your gut has been telling you for years that something doesn't fit -- if the treatments help but never hold, if the symptoms are strange in ways you've never been able to articulate clearly enough to get traction -- give the machines a chance to look.

The hope horizon isn't only in the research pipeline. It's already in your hands.

A Snapshot of the Pipeline: The Next Wave of Weapons

Think of the migraine treatments we have now as the revolutionary first-generation iPhone. It changed everything. But the technology we're about to discuss? This is the iPhone 17 Pro Max. It's faster, smarter, more efficient, and has features we couldn't have dreamed of just a few years ago.

The future of migraine solutions:

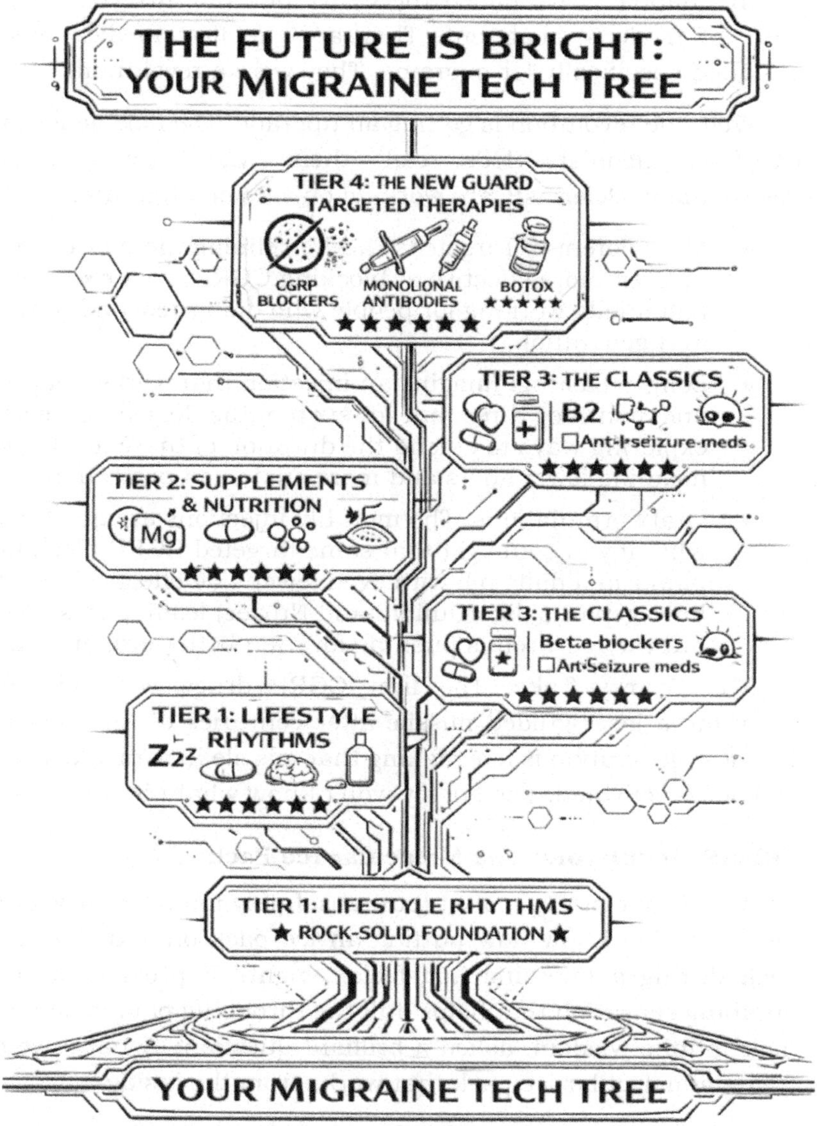

This image was created with the help of AI.

CGRP v2 Antagonists: The Smart Bomb Gets a Jetpack

In Chapter 7, we hailed the CGRP-blocking drugs as the rock stars of modern treatment. They are the first medications ever designed specifically for migraine. They were a revolution.

Well, the revolution is getting an upgrade. The next generation of CGRP antagonists---let's call them v2.0---are already in development. Scientists are working on versions that are:

- More Potent & Targeted: They're refining the molecules to be even more effective at blocking CGRP or its receptor, potentially working for people who didn't respond to the first generation.
- Longer-Lasting: Imagine an injection that works not just for one month or three, but for six months. Researchers are exploring ways to extend the duration of these antibodies, meaning fewer shots and more sustained protection.
- Oral Formulations: The monthly injections are great, but what if you could get that same targeted CGRP-blocking power in a daily pill with even fewer side effects? We already have gepants (like Qulipta and Nurtec) leading this charge, but the research is pushing for even better oral options.

The Snarky Take: The first CGRP drugs were like finally inventing a laser-guided missile after centuries of throwing rocks. The next generation is like making that missile hypersonic, invisible, and voice-activated. The enemy won't know what hit it.

TRPM8 Modulators: The Molecular Ice Pack

This is one of the coolest (pun absolutely intended) new areas of research. You know how putting an ice pack on your forehead or neck during a migraine just feels... right? It provides a cooling, numbing sensation that helps dull the throbbing pain. Scientists, in their infinite wisdom, asked a brilliant question: "What if we could create a molecular ice pack that works from the inside?"

That's where the TRPM8 (Transient Receptor Potential Melastatin 8) channel comes in. This is a protein found on your nerve endings that acts as the body's primary cold and menthol sensor. When you feel a cool breeze or apply a menthol-based rub, it's the TRPM8 channel firing up and sending that "cold" signal to your brain.

Here's the magic: when you activate the TRPM8 channel, it can actually inhibit the activity of other nearby pain-sensing nerves, like the ones that are screaming during a migraine. It's a phenomenon called neural cross-talk. By turning on the "cold" signal, you can effectively turn down the volume of the "pain" signal.

Researchers are now developing drugs (modulators) that can directly activate this TRPM8 channel. The idea is to have a pill or a nasal spray that could provide that deep, internal cooling and pain-inhibiting sensation without you ever having to touch a frozen bag of peas again.

The Snarky Take: This is science at its absolute finest. It's taking the most primal, desperate thing we do during an attack---slapping something cold on our head---and turning it into high-tech pharmacology. It's the ultimate "Hold my beer, I can do this better" moment from the scientific community.

Wearable EEG Predictors: A Weather Forecast for Your Brain

This is where we enter true sci-fi territory. For years, the holy grail of migraine management has been prediction. What if you could know an attack was coming hours before you even felt the first prodrome symptom?

Enter wearable EEG (electroencephalography) predictors.

EEG is a technology that measures the electrical activity of your brain---your brainwaves. We know that in the hours leading up to a migraine attack, the brain's electrical patterns begin to change in subtle but detectable ways. The problem has always been that EEG required a cumbersome cap with dozens of electrodes and a visit to a hospital.

Not anymore. Companies are now developing sleek, discreet, and comfortable headbands or patches that you can wear while you sleep or work. These devices use advanced sensors to continuously monitor your brainwaves. Their powerful AI algorithms learn your brain's unique pre-migraine electrical signature.

When the device detects those tell-tale changes, it will send an alert directly to your smartphone: "Neurological Storm Advisory: High probability of a migraine attack within the next 3-6 hours. Deploy countermeasures now."

This is not a guess. This is a forecast based on your own real-time brain data. It's the ultimate early-warning system. It gives you the power to pre-emptively medicate, hydrate, cancel plans, and get to your dark room before the first horseman even saddles up.

The Snarky Take: This is basically a weather app for the climate inside your skull. Instead of telling you if you need an umbrella, it tells you if you need a triptan and a sick note for work. It's the closest we'll ever get to having a migraine-psychic on retainer.

Beyond the Big Three: Other Exciting Avenues

The pipeline is deeper than just those three headliners. Scientists are attacking migraine from every conceivable angle, leading to some other incredibly promising areas of research.

PACAP Inhibitors: Targeting CGRP's Evil Twin

- What It Is: For years, CGRP got all the attention. But it turns out, it has a co-conspirator called PACAP (Pituitary Adenylate Cyclase-Activating Polypeptide). PACAP is another signaling molecule that is released during a migraine attack and contributes to the pain and inflammation. For some people---especially those who don't respond well to CGRP blockers---PACAP might be the primary driver of their attacks.
- The Future: Researchers are now developing drugs that specifically block PACAP or its receptors. This is the next level of personalized medicine. Imagine a future where your doctor can say, "Okay, the CGRP drugs didn't work for you, which suggests you might be a 'PACAP-dominant' migraineur. Let's try this instead." It's a whole new playbook for a whole new subset of warriors.
- The Snarky Take: It turns out the main villain might have a sidekick who is sometimes even more destructive. Science is now developing a weapon specifically for him, too. We're coming for the whole syndicate.

Digital Therapeutics (DTx): The Prescription on Your Phone

- What It Is: Get ready for a new category of medicine: prescription digital therapeutics. This isn't a wellness app you download for free. This is a clinically-tested, FDA-cleared software program that a doctor prescribes to you, just like a pill.

- How it Works: These apps deliver therapeutic interventions directly to the patient. For migraine, this could be a structured, interactive program that delivers Cognitive Behavioral Therapy (CBT) to help you manage the anxiety loop, biofeedback to teach you how to regulate your physiological stress response, or targeted coaching to help you identify triggers and modify your lifestyle. One such therapeutic, CT-132, has already been granted Breakthrough Device designation by the FDA.
- The Snarky Take: Your doctor is going to prescribe you... an app. Your phone, the device that has likely contributed to your eye strain and tech neck, is about to become a legitimate medical device. What a time to be alive.

How Clinical Trials Work (and Why You Should Consider Being a Hero)

All of this science gets from the lab to your medicine cabinet through one process: clinical trials.

And the only way clinical trials happen is with volunteers. With people like you.

I know what you're thinking. "Guinea pig." "Experiment." "What if I get a sugar pill?" The perception of clinical trials is often shrouded in mystery and fear. Let's pull back the curtain and demystify the process, because participating in a trial isn't just about being a test subject; it's about being a pioneer.

Busting the Myths: What a Modern Trial Is Actually Like

Myth #1: "I'll be a guinea pig for some untested, dangerous drug."

- Reality: By the time a drug reaches human trials, it has already gone through years of extensive laboratory and animal testing to ensure it's safe for initial study. Furthermore, trials are conducted in carefully controlled phases to maximize safety. You are monitored more closely by top-tier medical staff during a clinical trial than at any other time in your healthcare journey.

Myth #2: "They'll just give me a placebo (a sugar pill) and let me suffer."

- Reality: This is the biggest fear, and it's mostly outdated. While some trials do use a placebo group, it is considered increasingly unethical to deny treatment to people with a serious, painful condition. In most modern migraine trials, especially for prevention, the comparison is often between the new drug and the current best standard of care, or the new drug added on top of your existing regimen. And even if you are in a placebo group, the trial is usually short-term, and you are often offered access to the real drug after the trial ends (in what's called an open-label extension).

Myth #3: "It's a huge, complicated commitment."

- Reality: It is a commitment, but the research team makes it as easy as possible. They will walk you through every single step. All your appointments, tests, and the medication itself are provided free of charge. You are often compensated for your time and travel. And most importantly, you have the right to leave the trial at any time, for any reason, with no penalty.

The Four Phases of a Clinical Trial (The Journey from Lab to Pharmacy)

Understanding the process can help reduce the fear. Here's the typical journey a new drug takes:

- Phase I: Is it Safe? The new drug is given to a very small group of healthy volunteers (not patients) to test for basic safety, dosage, and side effects.
- Phase II: Does it Work? The drug is given to a slightly larger group of people who actually have the condition (e.g., migraine warriors) to see if it has the desired effect and to further evaluate its safety and dosage.
- Phase III: Is it Better Than What We Have? This is the big one. The drug is given to a large group of patients (hundreds or thousands) and is compared against a placebo or the current standard treatment. This is the final, rigorous test to prove its effectiveness and safety before it can be submitted to the FDA for approval.
- Phase IV: What Happens in the Real World? After the drug is approved and on the market, these studies continue to monitor its long-term effectiveness and safety in a broad, real-world population.

Why You Should Genuinely Consider It

There are two main reasons to participate in a clinical trial, and they are both incredibly powerful.

- For Everyone Else (The Altruistic Reason): You become a hero. It is not an exaggeration to say that every single medication you take, from a simple aspirin to a complex biologic, exists because people before you volunteered for a clinical trial. They endured the uncertainty so that you could have a proven treatment. Participating is your chance to pay it forward. You are actively contributing to the advancement of science and helping to create a better future for millions of fellow migraine sufferers, including generations to come. You are not just a patient; you are a partner in discovery.
- For You (The Self-Interested Reason): You get access to the future, right now. You have the opportunity to receive a potentially life-changing, cutting-edge treatment years before it becomes available to the general public. You will also receive expert medical care from leading specialists in the field, often at no cost to you. For someone who has tried and failed multiple other treatments, a clinical trial can be a source of profound new hope and a very real chance at relief.

CALL-TO-ACTION BOX: How to Find a Clinical Trial Near You

Ready to go from warrior to pioneer? Finding a trial is easier than you think. Here's your toolkit.

1. The Master Database: ClinicalTrials.gov

- This is the official, comprehensive registry of clinical trials run by the U.S. National Library of Medicine. It is the most trustworthy source.

How to Use It:

Go to www.clinicaltrials.gov.

In the "Condition or disease" search box, type in "Migraine" or "Headache."

- In the "Country" field, select your country. In the "City, State" field, enter your location to find trials near you.
- You can use the filters to narrow your search by trial phase, age group, and more.

2. Advocacy Group Resources:

- Organizations like the American Migraine Foundation and the National Headache Foundation often have their own user-friendly trial finders or lists of recruiting studies. They are a great place to look.

3. Talk to Your Doctor:

- Your neurologist or headache specialist is often aware of recruiting trials in your area. Ask them directly.
- Your Script: "I'm interested in exploring all my options, and I'd like to learn more about participating in migraine research. Are you aware of any clinical trials in this area that I might be a good candidate for?"

Conclusion: The Future is a Verb

Hope is a powerful thing. But for a long time, hope in the migraine world felt passive---a wish, a prayer, a distant dream that maybe, someday, things would get better.

What the science and research on the horizon tell us is that hope is no longer a noun. It's a verb. It is something we can actively participate in. The future of migraine treatment isn't something that is happening to us; it's something that is happening because of us. Because of the warriors who raise their hands to join a trial, who meticulously track their data in an app, who advocate for more research funding, and who share their stories to fight stigma.

And -- I would add one more thing to that list -- because of the patients who refuse to accept an incomplete answer. Who keep asking questions when the treatment works but doesn't hold. Who upload old scans at midnight because they still believe there is something to find. Who trust their own bodies enough to push back on a narrative that fits most of their symptoms but not all of them.

The pace of innovation is real. The breakthroughs are happening. The brilliant minds are hard at work. We are on the cusp of an era of truly personalized, targeted, and effective migraine care. A future where our children might know migraine only as a condition that was once debilitating, but is now easily managed.

And the tools being built in that future -- the AI assistants, the diagnostic models, the pattern-recognition systems -- are not just for researchers and clinicians. They are for you. They are for the patient sitting alone at 1 AM with a stack of imaging reports and a question nobody in the system has fully answered yet.

Here is the one thing I want you to do after reading this chapter.

You don't have to enroll in a trial tomorrow. You don't have to donate your life savings to research. You just have to do one thing.

Open your web browser and click the link: ClinicalTrials.gov.

Spend five minutes just looking. See the names of the new drugs being tested. See the universities and hospitals that are leading the charge. See the sheer volume of work that is being done, right now, on your behalf.

That is what hope looks like. It's not a fantasy. It's a dataset. It's a clinical trial entry. It's the relentless, brilliant, and unstoppable march of science. It's an AI reading a scan at midnight and changing one person's life. Go take a look. Knowledge is hope. Go get some.

Conclusion:

Here it is. The end of the line. The final chapter. The part where the hero, bruised and battered but standing tall, looks back at the battlefield and takes stock of how far they've come.

I started this book in the middle of my own story, not the end of it, and I want to close it the same way—honestly. The structural source of my pain has been identified. Diagnostic injections confirmed it. As I write this, surgery is on the horizon. I don't know how my story ends yet. Nobody does, while they're living it. What I know is that I no longer wonder what's wrong with me. I have a name for it, a mechanism that explains it, and a path forward that makes sense. And the thing that gave me the thread—after five years and eight doctors—was refusing to stop asking questions, and being willing to use every tool available, including ones that didn't exist when my journey started.

I wrote this book during the part of the journey where I was still in the dark but starting to find the edges of the light. That felt like exactly where it needed to come from. You deserve an answer. Keep looking until you find it.

But before I send you off, take a moment. Put the book down and take a deep breath (as long as deep breathing isn't a trigger). You've just completed a masterclass in your own neurology.

This isn't a fluffy wrap-up where we all feel good for three minutes and then go back to our regularly scheduled misery. This is your graduation.

You didn't just read a book. You went to war college.

You picked up this guide as a patient, maybe even as a victim---a person to whom migraines happened. You were a hostage to the whims of your own brain, living in a state of constant, low-grade fear, just waiting for the next attack to derail your life.

But you're not that person anymore.

Look at what you've done. Look at what you now know. You are an entirely different kind of warrior now. So, before we send you off into the world armed with your new arsenal of knowledge and snark, let's recap the epic journey you just completed. Let's review the superhero origin story you just wrote for yourself.

You understand the Four Horsemen. You can identify your enemy in the Migraine Multiverse, read the script of an attack before Act III lands, track the domino conspiracy of your triggers, and walk into a doctor's office with data instead of desperation. You have an acute playbook, a preventive arsenal, a hacked habitat, a communication strategy, and a full Field Manual in your back pocket. You know when your "migraine" might be something else entirely—and you know how to push until you get a real answer.

That is not nothing. That is everything.

The New You: From Victim to Warrior-Strategist

Look back at that list. That is your new resume.

The person who started this book was likely living in a reactive state, tossed about by the unpredictable waves of their condition. The person who has finished this book is a proactive, data-driven, self-aware expert.

You have fundamentally changed your relationship with your migraines. You no longer see them as a mysterious curse, but as a complex biological process that you understand and can influence. You have moved from a place of fear to a place of strategy. You have traded helplessness for empowerment.

This is not about being "cured." I have never and will never promise you a cure. The world of chronic illness is rarely that simple. There will still be bad days. There will still be attacks that break through your defenses. There will still be pain.

But here is the crucial difference: you will never again be unprepared.

When the next attack comes, you will not be a surprised victim. You will be a prepared warrior executing a well-rehearsed plan. You will know what's happening in your brain, you will know what phase you're in, and you will know exactly what tools to deploy. You will have your Code Red Kit ready. You will have your dark room prepped. You will have your guilt-free scripts ready to send.

And on the good days, you will not be living in fear of the next attack. You will be actively building your fortress. You will be prioritizing your sleep, managing your stress, hacking your environment, and advocating for your health.

The pain may still come, but the suffering---the suffering that comes from fear, from misunderstanding, from guilt, from helplessness---that part of the battle is already won. You have dismantled it, piece by piece, with knowledge and strategy.

A Final Dose of Snarky Realism

Let's be clear. You are now armed with an arsenal of information that would make a first-year neurology resident sweat. But knowledge is not a magic shield. Life will still happen.

Your boss will still schedule a last-minute, high-stress meeting. Your kid will still get a stomach bug in the middle of the night, wrecking your perfect sleep schedule. A thunderstorm will still roll in and send the barometric pressure plummeting. Your hormones will still do their chaotic monthly dance.

You will still get migraines.

The goal was never to create a perfect, trigger-free life. That's a fantasy that only serves to make us feel like failures. The goal was to build resilience. It was to give you so many tools, so many strategies, and so much knowledge that you can handle the inherent chaos of life without it inevitably leading to a neurological collapse.

It's about knowing that when the dominoes start to fall---and they will fall---you now have the power to pull one or two out of the chain before they all come crashing down. It's about turning a catastrophic 10/10 migraine into a manageable 5/10 day. It's about reducing your 15 migraine days a month to five. It's about reclaiming the 80% of your life that was being held hostage by the other 20%.

That is a victory worth fighting for.

Your Final Mission: Pass the Torch

And now, for your final piece of actionable advice. Your graduation assignment.

Through this entire book, you have been a student, absorbing information and turning inward to understand your own experience. Your final mission is to turn that knowledge outward. The final stage of mastery is not just knowing; it's teaching.

Your mission is this: Pick one thing. Just one single, powerful truth you've learned from this book, and share it.

This is your call to action. It can be big or small, public or private.

- Maybe you sit down with your partner and finally walk them through the Care-Partner One-Pager. You give them the gift of knowing how to help.

Maybe you send the Template Email for HR Accommodations to your boss, finally advocating for the workspace you deserve.

- Maybe you see another migraine sufferer posting in an online forum about their guilt over missing a family event, and you share the Guilt-Spiral Interrupt Protocol with them.
- Maybe you just have a calm, confident conversation with your well-meaning Aunt Karen, using the "my doctor and I have a plan" script to finally shut down the celery juice conversation.
- Maybe you just explain to a friend, using the Four Horsemen analogy, why your migraine is not just a headache.

Why is this your final mission? Because the moment you successfully explain a piece of this to someone else, something shifts. You stop being someone who only absorbs information and become a source of it. You are an advocate. You are a beacon for others who are still lost in the dark.

By sharing your knowledge, you fight the stigma that keeps so many of us suffering in silence. You empower the people around you to be better allies. And you solidify, in your own mind, the new reality: You are in control.

♥□ A Final Word to Everyone in the Room

To the partners, parents, children, friends, managers, and anyone else who picked up this book trying to understand someone they love:

You made it to the end. That tells me everything I need to know about you.

The fact that you read this -- that you wanted to understand the Four Horsemen, the Trigger Matrix, the guilt spiral, the specialist referrals, the insurance appeals -- means you are not a bystander. You are part of the solution. And that matters more than you know.

Living with chronic pain is isolating in a specific and particular way. Not because the people around you don't care. They do. But because the condition is invisible and unpredictable and hard to explain, and because the person in pain often spends enormous energy trying not to be a burden. They cancel plans with an apology rather than an explanation. They push through when they should rest, because they're afraid of disappointing you. They downplay how bad it is, because they've told you how bad it is before and they can see the helplessness in your face, and they can't bear to put that there again.

What you can give them -- the most powerful thing, actually -- is not fixes. It's witness.

You don't have to solve it. You can't. Nobody can, fully. What you can do is show up, consistently and without resentment, and make it clear that you are still there. That the bad days don't scare you away. That canceled plans are genuinely forgiven, not just tolerated. That the darkened room and the ice pack and the silence are things you understand now, even a little, because you took the time to read a book about it.

That is not a small thing. That is, for many people living with chronic pain, the difference between enduring and belonging.

So here is what I want to ask you to do -- just one thing, the same final assignment the migraine warrior reading this is getting:

Pick one thing you learned from this book and use it.

Maybe you set up the Care-Partner One-Pager on your phone so you have it for the next attack. Maybe you stop asking "are you okay?" during an attack and start just quietly handling whatever you can handle. Maybe you tell your person -- out loud, or in a text -- that you read this and you understand more than you did before, and you're not going anywhere.

That's it. You don't have to be perfect. You just have to show up.

The person in your life with migraines is working very hard, every day, to hold their life together around something that keeps trying to pull it apart. They are braver and more resilient than they know. And they are better -- calmer, more grounded, more capable of handling the hard days -- because you are in their corner.

Thank you for being there. It matters.

A Final Word: The Warrior's Send-Off

You did it. You walked through the fire, and you came out the other side not just unscathed, but forged into something stronger.

Remember that you are not alone. There is a vast, global army of us---millions strong---fighting this same battle every single day. We are in every office, every school, every family. We are the ones wearing sunglasses indoors, sipping water religiously, and silently cheering when someone else understands. We are your community. Welcome to the club. It's a crappy club, but the people in it are some of the most resilient, empathetic, and badass warriors you will ever meet.

So go. Take this knowledge. Use your tools. Hack your habitat. Advocate for yourself with the fierce confidence of a CEO. And on the hard days, when the pain comes and the darkness descends, remember the army that stands with you.

And know this: you are doing so much better than you think you are.

Now, go live your life. You've earned it.

FIELD MANUAL (The Appendix)

Your Tear-Out, Post-on-the-Fridge, Quick-Reference Toolkit

Six tools. Tear them out, screenshot them, post them on your fridge. These are built for the moments when brain fog has stolen your memory or a loved one is staring at you asking "What do I do?" This is a section you use, not just read.

- A. The Migraine Phase Wheel: Your at-a-glance diagnostic tool to figure out where you are in an attack and what your immediate next move is.
- B. The Trigger Matrix Poster: Your advanced detective's wall, for tracking the complex conspiracies your triggers are plotting against you.
- C. The Medication Family Tree: Your visual guide to the pharmaceutical arsenal, helping you understand the weapons your doctor might recommend.
- D. The Care-Partner One-Pager: The emergency instruction manual you can shove into the hands of a loved one when you can no longer form coherent sentences.
- E. The Doctor Visit Planner: The ultimate pre-mission briefing sheet to ensure you walk out of every doctor's appointment with a clear plan, not just a confused look and another bill.
- F. The AI Diagnostic Tool Quick-Reference Card: For when you've done everything right and still don't have a complete answer -- a step-by-step guide to using AI tools to review your imaging and medical history as a diagnostic supplement.

This is your gear. Learn it. Use it. Own it. Welcome to the armory. Let's get you equipped.

This is your tactical command center for an active migraine attack. In the fog of war, it's easy to forget the script. This wheel is your pocket-sized director, reminding you what's happening, what's coming next, and what you need to do right now. Print this out and stick it somewhere you can see it every day. When you feel an attack coming on, find your phase on the wheel and execute the plan.

The Migraine Phase Wheel:

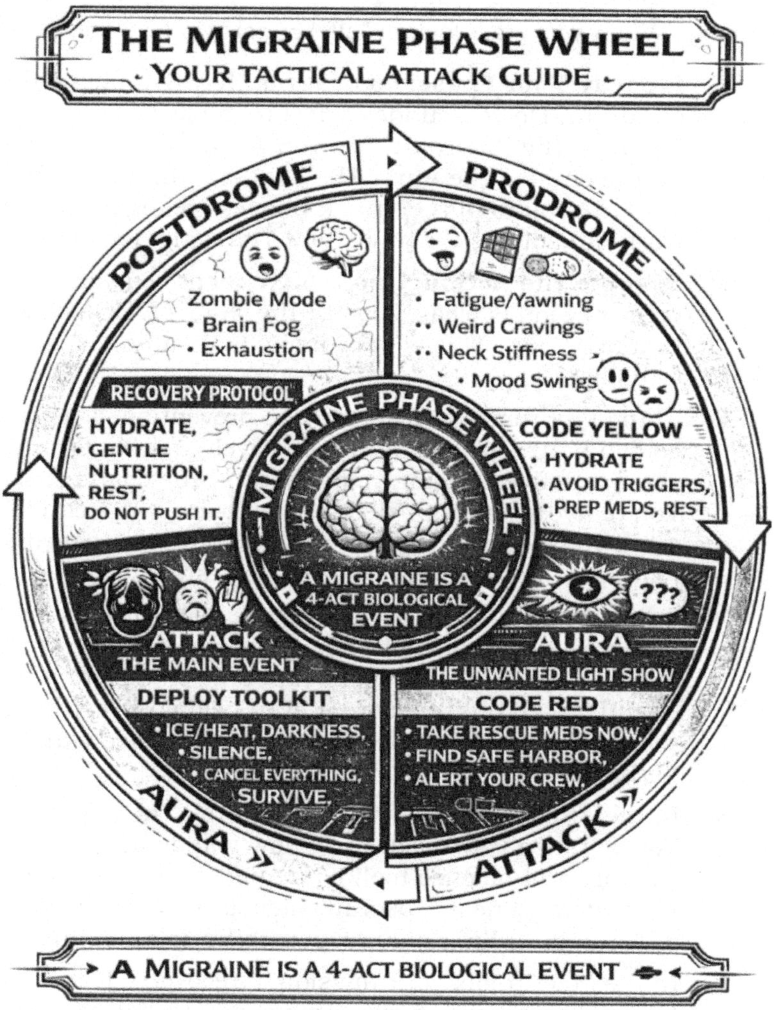

This image was created with the help of AI.

How to Use Your Phase Wheel:

The Phase Wheel is your "You Are Here" map for the migraine journey. When you start feeling "off," consult the wheel.

- **Identify Your Phase:** Look at the "Key Symptoms" in each quadrant. Do you suddenly feel irritable and crave salt? You're in the Prodrome. Are you seeing shimmering lights? You've entered the Aura. The head-splitting throb has started? You're in the Attack phase. Feeling like a foggy, worn-out zombie the day after? That's the Postdrome.
- **Execute the Action:** Once you've identified your phase, your mission is clear. Look at the "KEY ACTION" box for that quadrant. This is your immediate, no-questions-asked to-do list.
- In the Prodrome, your mission is prevention. This is your golden hour. You're not just passively waiting for the pain; you are actively taking steps to blunt the coming assault. You're hydrating with electrolytes, being extra careful to avoid your known triggers, getting your rescue medications ready just in case, and prioritizing rest.
- In the Aura, your mission is interception. The moment it starts, you have one job: take your fastest-acting rescue medication. This is your one and only chance to potentially stop the pain phase before it even begins. Everything else is secondary. Get to a safe place, take your meds, and prepare for battle.
- In the Attack, your mission is survival. The battle is here. You've taken your meds, and now you deploy your full comfort-and-defense toolkit. Ice packs, heating pads, absolute darkness, absolute silence. You cancel your plans without guilt. Your only responsibility is to endure.
- In the Postdrome, your mission is recovery. This is not the time to "catch up" on everything you missed. Your brain is a battlefield under repair. Pushing yourself now is like trying to run a marathon on a sprained ankle---you're just asking for another injury (i.e., another migraine). Your job is to gently refuel with good nutrition and hydration, and to rest as much as humanly possible.

This wheel turns the chaos of an attack into a predictable sequence of events. When you know what's coming, you are no longer a victim of the chaos. You are the strategist who is one step ahead.

B. The Trigger Matrix Poster

Your standard migraine diary is great for logging individual attacks. But where it often fails is in showing you the complex conspiracies---the way your triggers team up and work together. The Trigger Matrix is your detective's conspiracy board. It helps you see, at a glance, how the dominoes fell over the course of a week.

This isn't about just finding a single trigger. It's about finding your personal recipe for disaster. Maybe it's not just the red wine, but the red wine plus a poor night's sleep plus a stressful Wednesday. This matrix will help you see that pattern.

Print a new copy of the blank matrix every Sunday. Fill it out each evening before bed. At the end of the week, put it up on your wall and look for connections.

The Trigger Matrix:

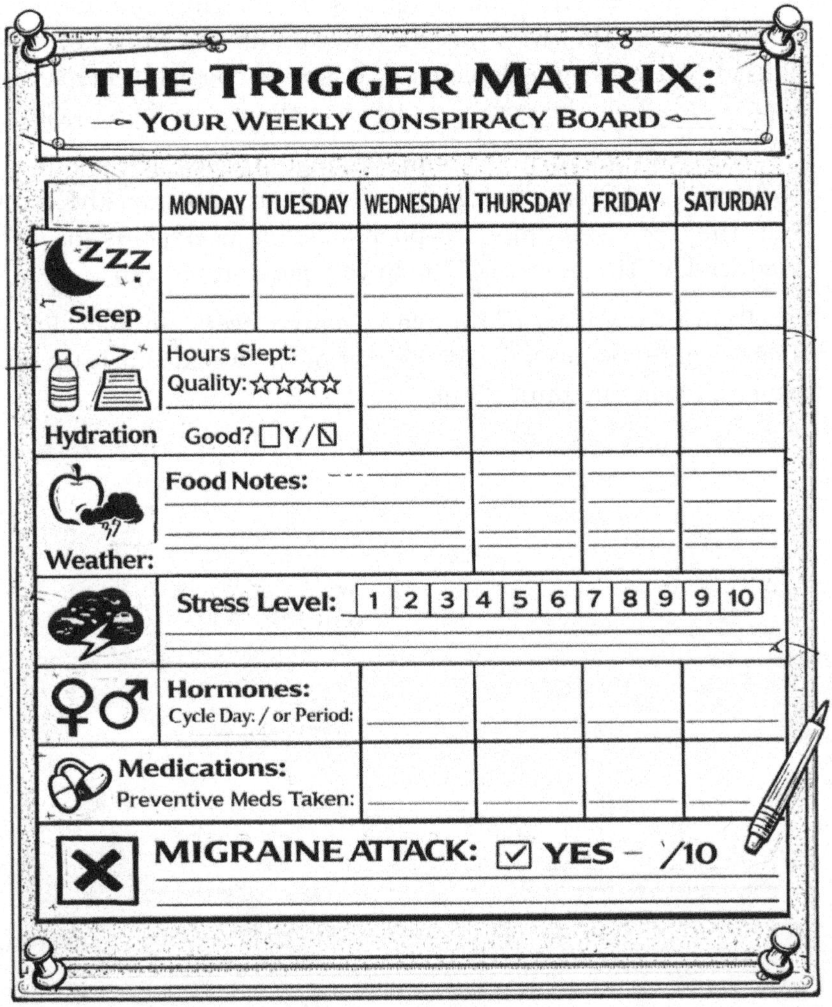

This image was created with the help of AI.

How to Use Your Trigger Matrix:

- The Daily Debrief: Every evening, take 60 seconds to fill out the column for that day. Be honest. Did you really drink enough water? Was your stress level truly a 2 or was it more like a 7? The more accurate your data, the more powerful your insights will be.
- Mark the Attack: If you had a migraine attack that day, put a big, angry checkmark or "X" in the bottom box and note the peak pain level. This is the "crime" we are trying to solve.
- The Weekly Review (The Detective Work): At the end of the week, look at your completed matrix. Look at the column where the migraine attack happened. Now, look up that column at all the other factors on that day. More importantly, look at the column for the day before. This is where the conspiracies are revealed.

Let's Analyze the Sample Matrix:

Let's say our sample warrior, let's call him Bob, had a brutal 8/10 migraine on Thursday. A quick look might make him blame the stressful presentation he had on Thursday afternoon. But with the matrix, he can see the whole conspiracy.

Thursday (Attack Day): Stress Level: 9/10. Hydration: Poor. Food: Skipped lunch.

- Wednesday (The Day Before): Sleep: Only 4 hours. Food Notes: "Late pizza and two beers." Weather: "Big storm rolled in."
- The Conspiracy Uncovered: The stressful presentation on Thursday wasn't the lone gunman. It was just the final domino. The real plot was hatched on Wednesday. Bob started Thursday with a massive sleep deficit (Brick 1), likely dehydrated from the beer (Brick 2), and with his system already on edge from the drop in barometric pressure (Brick 3). He was already standing on the edge of his migraine threshold. Skipping lunch and heading into a stressful meeting was all it took to push him over.

See the power? Bob's takeaway isn't "I need to avoid stress." That's impossible. His actionable takeaway is, "When I know I have a stressful day coming up, I absolutely must prioritize getting a full night's sleep and staying hydrated the day before. Those are the dominoes I can actually control."

This matrix gives you that power. It helps you stop blaming the final trigger and start defending against the first one.

C. The Medication Family Tree

Navigating the world of migraine medications can feel like trying to learn a foreign language while your head is on fire. Triptans, Gepants, CGRP Monoclonals, Beta-Blockers---what does it all mean? It's confusing, and it's easy to feel lost.

This Medication Family Tree is your visual translator. It's designed to help you understand the different "families" of drugs your doctor might discuss, how they work, and what to expect. This isn't a substitute for medical advice, but it is a powerful tool to help you have a more informed conversation about your options. Knowledge is power, especially when it comes to the complex chemistry of your own treatment plan.

Medication Family Tree:

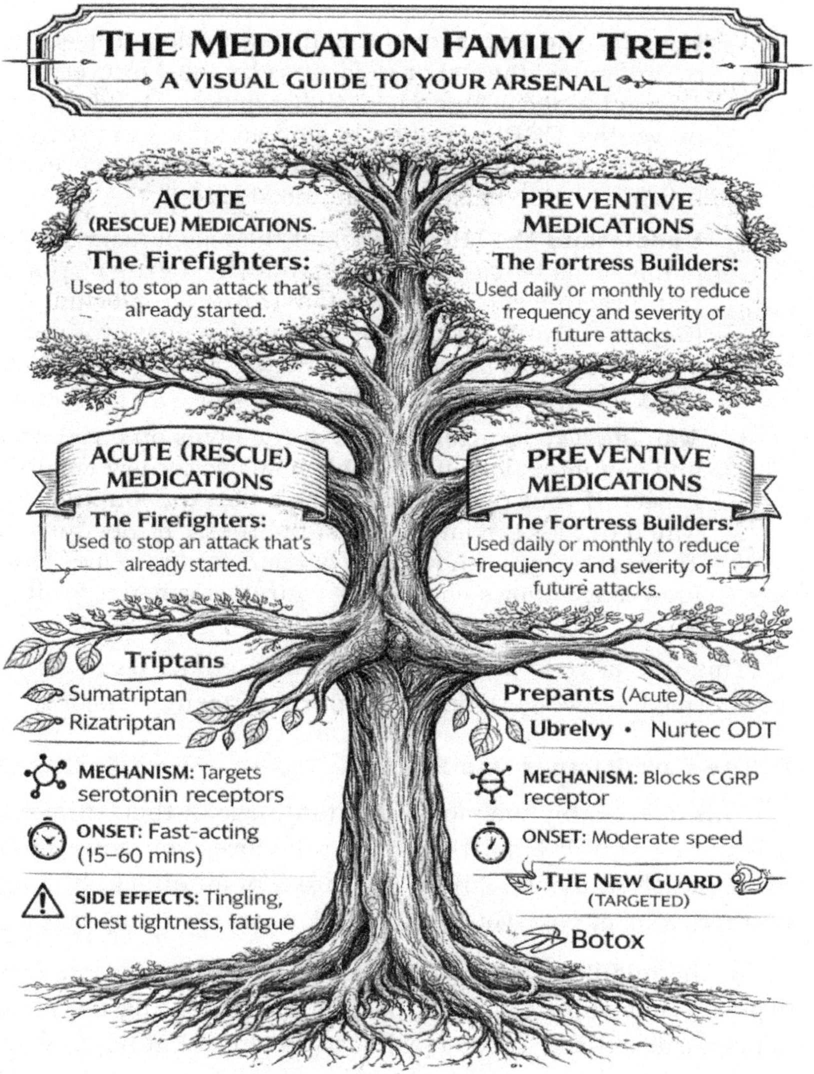
THE MEDICATION FAMILY TREE:
A VISUAL GUIDE TO YOUR ARSENAL
ACUTE
(RESCUE) MEDICATIONS
The Firefighters:
Used to stop an attack that's already started.
PREVENTIVE
MEDICATIONS
The Fortress Builders:
Used daily or monthly to reduce frequency and severity of future attacks.
ACUTE (RESCUE)
MEDICATIONS
The Firefighters:
Used to stop an attack that's already started.
PREVENTIVE
MEDICATIONS
The Fortress Builders:
Used daily or monthly to reduce frequency and severity of future attacks.
Triptans
Sumatriptan
Rizatriptan
MECHANISM: Targets serotonin receptors
ONSET: Fast-acting (15–60 mins)
SIDE EFFECTS: Tingling, chest tightness, fatigue
Prepants (Acute)
Ubrelvy • Nurtec ODT
MECHANISM: Blocks CGRP receptor
ONSET: Moderate speed
THE NEW GUARD
(TARGETED)
Botox

This image was created with the help of AI.

How to Use Your Medication Family Tree:

This tree helps you visualize where your current (or potential) medications fit into the grand scheme of things.

- **Identify the Purpose:** Is the drug your doctor is suggesting a "firefighter" (Acute) or a "fortress builder" (Preventive)? This is the most fundamental distinction. You don't use a preventive CGRP injection to stop an attack in progress, and you don't use an acute triptan every day to prevent future attacks (hello, rebound headaches).
- **Understand the "How":** Look at the mechanism for each family. This helps you understand why a drug works. Are you targeting serotonin (Triptans)? Are you blocking CGRP (Gepants, Antibodies)? Are you calming down your entire nervous system (Anti-Seizure Meds)? Knowing this helps you understand your doctor's strategy.
- **Manage Expectations:** Look at the notes on onset speed and common side effects. This helps you know what to expect. If your doctor prescribes a triptan, you know to watch out for tingling or chest tightness. If they prescribe Topiramate, you know to be on alert for brain fog. This knowledge allows you to give your doctor better feedback on how a medication is affecting you.

This tree is your pharmacological field guide. Use it to become an informed, active participant in your treatment decisions.

D. The Care-Partner One-Pager

This is arguably the most important page in this entire manual. It is not for you. It is for the person who loves you and who stands by helplessly while you are in the throes of an attack. It is for your partner, your parent, your best friend, or your roommate.

In the middle of a migraine, you can't communicate. You can't explain what you need. This page does the talking for you. It's a simple, calm, 5-step guide to what to do (and what not to do).

Our advice: In a moment of peace and calm, sit down with your primary care partner. Have them read this. Put it on the fridge or save a screenshot on their phone under "MIGRAINE EMERGENCY." When an attack hits, all you have to do is point. It removes the panic and helplessness for them, and the burden of communication for you.

How to help someone when they are experiencing a migraine:

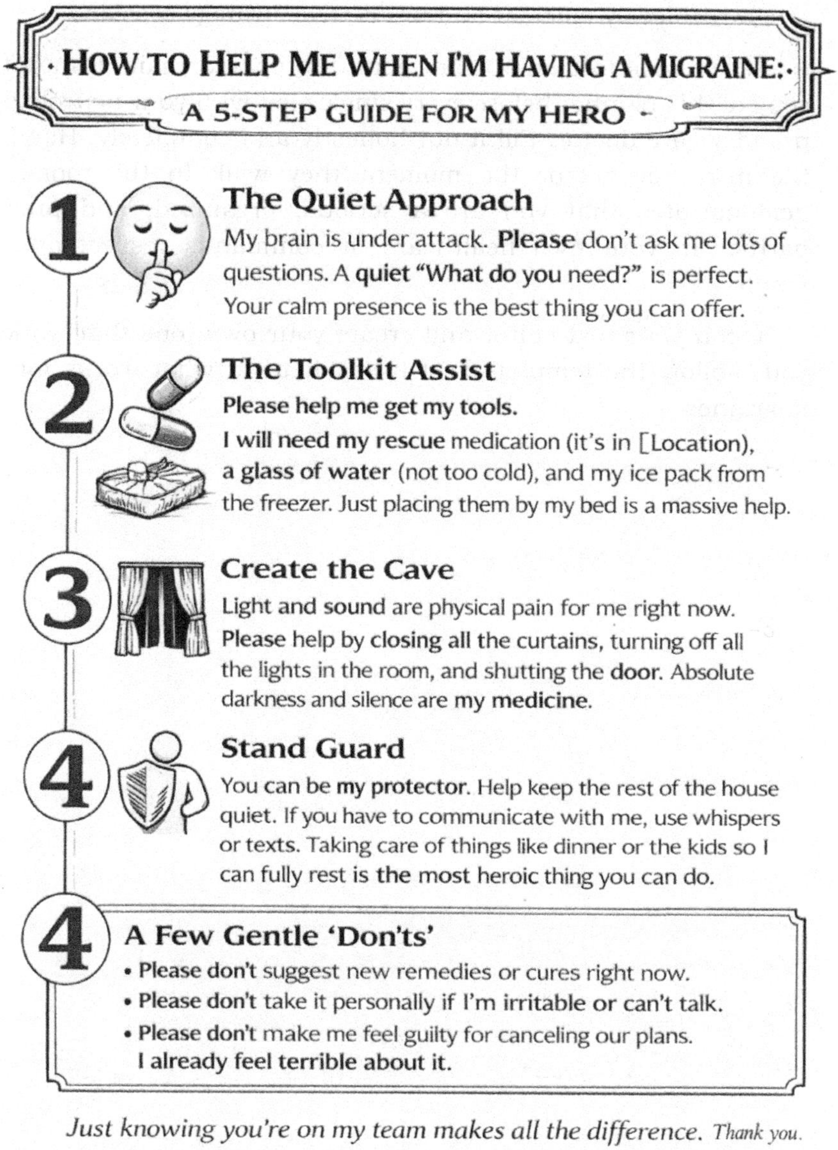

This image was created with the help of AI.

We introduced this concept in Chapter 11. This is the full, ready-to-use, fillable version of that tool. This single page is your key to transforming a rushed, confusing 15-minute doctor's appointment into a ruthlessly efficient and productive strategy session.

Never walk into an appointment unprepared again. Print a fresh copy of this planner before every single visit with your neurologist or primary care doctor. Fill it out honestly and completely. Hand it to the nurse or doctor the moment they walk in the room. This demonstrates that you are a serious, organized, and proactive partner in your own healthcare. It commands respect and gets results.

Open your text editor and create your own, one that works for you. Follow the template and tweak it to fit what works for your migraines.

How to help someone when they are experiencing a migraine:

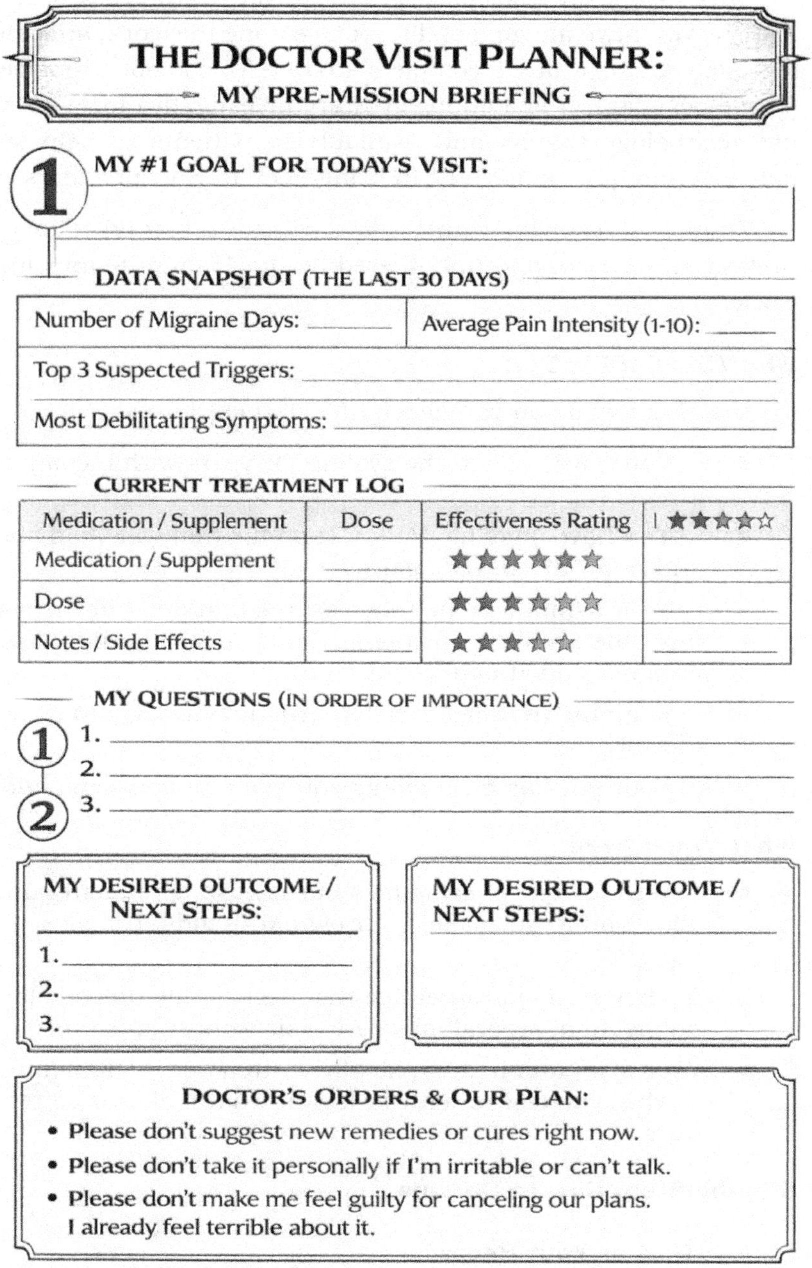

THE DOCTOR VISIT PLANNER:

MY PRE-MISSION BRIEFING

1 MY #1 GOAL FOR TODAY'S VISIT:

DATA SNAPSHOT (THE LAST 30 DAYS)

Number of Migraine Days: ______	Average Pain Intensity (1-10): ______
Top 3 Suspected Triggers: ______	
Most Debilitating Symptoms: ______	

CURRENT TREATMENT LOG

Medication / Supplement	Dose	Effectiveness Rating	I ★★★★☆
Medication / Supplement	______	★★★★★★	______
Dose	______	★★★★★★	______
Notes / Side Effects	______	★★★★★	______

MY QUESTIONS (IN ORDER OF IMPORTANCE)

1. ______
2. ______
3. ______

MY DESIRED OUTCOME / NEXT STEPS:

1. ______
2. ______
3. ______

MY DESIRED OUTCOME / NEXT STEPS:

DOCTOR'S ORDERS & OUR PLAN:

- Please don't suggest new remedies or cures right now.
- Please don't take it personally if I'm irritable or can't talk.
- Please don't make me feel guilty for canceling our plans. I already feel terrible about it.

This image was created with the help of AI.

F. The AI Diagnostic Tool Quick-Reference Card

This tool is for a specific situation: you have years of medical history, you have imaging on file, you've done the work, and you still feel like you don't have a complete answer. This is not a replacement for medical care. It is a supplementary investigative tool -- a way to use technology that is now available to patients to help surface patterns and questions you can bring back to your providers.

Think of it as giving your medical records a second set of eyes -- tireless, unhurried, and unbothered by the 15-minute appointment clock.

Who This Card Is For:

Use this tool if you can check ANY of these boxes:

- [ ] You have been in the system for years with incomplete answers
- [ ] You have imaging (MRI, CT) on file that was read once and never discussed again
- [ ] Your symptoms include features that don't fit the classic migraine profile -- positional changes, facial numbness, arm weakness, load-dependent pain
- [ ] Migraine treatments help partially but never fully or durably
- [ ] Your gut has been telling you something doesn't add up

What You'll Need

- Access to your imaging files (most hospital patient portals allow you to download your own MRI and CT images and reports)
- A current AI chat interface that accepts file uploads (as of publication, several major AI assistants support this)
- Your symptom history, ideally written out in plain language -- what you feel, when you feel it, what makes it better or worse

Step-by-Step: How to Do This

Step 1: Gather Your Records

Log into your patient portal and download:

- Any MRI or CT reports (the written radiology reads)

- The actual imaging files if the portal allows (DICOM format)
- Any neurology or specialist notes that summarize your diagnostic history

If you can't access digital files, call your radiology department and request your records. You have a legal right to them.

Step 2: Open an AI Assistant

Use a major, reputable AI assistant. You are not looking for a diagnosis. You are looking for a conversation that helps you understand what your records actually say and whether there are findings worth asking your doctor about.

Step 3: Upload and Ask Structured Questions

Start with the radiology report text (copy and paste, or upload the document). Then ask:

- "Can you walk me through the key findings in this radiology report in plain language?"
- "Are there any findings here that could be related to head pain or neurological symptoms?"
- "My symptoms include [list your specific symptoms]. Do any of the findings in this report potentially relate to those?"
- "Are there any findings mentioned here that a neurologist versus a spine specialist would typically evaluate?"

Then provide your symptom history and ask:

- "Given this symptom pattern and these imaging findings, what questions might be worth asking a doctor who hasn't seen both together?"

Step 4: Document What You Find

Write down or screenshot anything that feels significant. You are not diagnosing yourself. You are building a list of informed questions to bring back to your medical team.

Step 5: Bring It to a Provider

Take what you found -- the questions, the specific imaging references, the pattern you noticed -- and bring it to an appropriate specialist. Frame it as: "I was reviewing my old imaging and I wanted to ask whether [specific finding] might be contributing to my symptoms."

You are not telling them the AI diagnosed you. You are telling them you did your homework and you have a specific question. That is good advocacy. That is what this book has been training you to do.

Important Caveats (Read These)

AI tools make mistakes. They can misread context, miss nuance, or surface findings that are incidental and not clinically relevant to your symptoms. Nothing that comes out of this process is a diagnosis. It is a starting point for a conversation.

What AI does exceptionally well is pattern recognition across large amounts of text, without the time pressure and specialty tunnel vision that can affect human clinical encounters. It will read every word of your imaging report. It will not skip the fine print. It will ask follow-up questions you may not have thought to ask.

Use it as the tool it is: a tireless research assistant working for you, in service of a conversation you will have with a qualified human being who can actually examine you and make clinical judgments.

That human still matters. The tool just helps you show up to that conversation better prepared.

Conclusion: Your Arsenal is Complete

And there you have it. Your Field Manual is fully stocked. These six tools---the Phase Wheel, the Trigger Matrix, the Medication Family Tree, the Care-Partner One-Pager, the Doctor Visit Planner, and the AI Diagnostic Quick-Reference Card---are your tactical advantage.

They are designed to bring clarity to the chaos, to turn data into action, and to transform you and your loved ones from a scattered militia into a coordinated, elite fighting force.

But here's the most important thing: a weapon is useless if it stays locked in the armory. These tools are not meant to be admired. They are meant to be used until they are wrinkled, coffee-stained, and covered in your notes.

So, here is your final mission, your last piece of actionable homework. Pick one.

Just one of these tools. The one that made you think, "Oh, I need that." Is it the Doctor Planner for your appointment next month? Is it the One-Pager to finally give to your spouse? Is it the Trigger Matrix because you're ready to get serious about your detective work? Is it the AI card because you have a stack of old imaging and a question that's never been fully answered?

Pick one. Print it out. Put it into action this week.

You are no longer just surviving. You are not just fighting back. With these tools in hand, you are strategizing, you are leading, and you are taking control. You are the architect, the detective, and the five-star general of your own well-being. Now, go win the war.

About the Author

Ken Konet, M.Ed., MBA

Ken Konet has three master's degrees, which sounds incredibly impressive until you realize that two of them are in fields that still couldn't help him figure out why his head hurt so much. He holds graduate degrees from Oxford University (yes, that Oxford—he checked twice to make sure it wasn't a typo), John Carroll University (a Jesuit institution in Cleveland where they apparently gave him a diploma despite his persistent tendency to question everything), and a third that rounds out what his friends generously call "a well-rounded overachiever problem."

By day, Ken is a Corporate Instructional Designer with deep experience in enterprise systems and workplace learning. He has spent his career making complicated things understandable—which, as it turns out, is exactly the skill set required to write a book about a neurological condition that most people still think is "just a simple headache."

Ken is also a prolific author across multiple genres, proving that the inside of his head is apparently a very busy place even while it's in pain.

He lives in Florida with his wife Izzy, who runs her own thriving handywoman business and is, by all accounts, both the more practical and more patient of the two. She tolerated years of cancelled plans, darkened rooms, and Ken's increasingly elaborate theories about what was wrong with his head—and then, when he finally figured it out with the help of AI, she was the one helping him haul equipment and furniture, which is how the cervical loading research got field-tested in the most inconvenient way possible.

Ken wrote this book from the middle of his own migraine story—not after it was resolved, but while he was still in it. He believes that's exactly where it needed to come from.

He is still looking forward to crawling under a car, working on the house, or going camping without paying for it for three days.

About the Clinical Contributor

Elliott James, APRN, MSN, CMRD

Elliott James has had an interest in brain science since he was a kid — which, in retrospect, makes him exactly the kind of person you want managing your neurological care. He earned his first Bachelor's degree at Stetson University, where he was studying behavioral neuroscience and working in the neuroscience lab of the psychology department. His senior research in Psychology was accepted and presented at the 2004 Southeastern Psychology Association conference in Nashville, Tennessee — which means he was doing actual neuroscience before most of us even knew what a neuron was.

He decided to go into healthcare always with the intention of working in Neurology — because apparently some people just know what they want to do with their lives, and the rest of us are deeply envious. He received a Bachelor's in Nursing from the University of Central Florida, and a Master's degree in Family Nurse Practitioner from Maryville University in St. Louis, Missouri.

Within Neurology, Elliott has a special interest in movement disorders, and in February 2025 earned a certification in movement and related disorders through the Association of Movement Disorder Advanced Practice Providers. The CMRD after his name isn't just alphabet soup — it means he has specialized, board-level expertise in the neurological conditions that make your body do things you didn't ask it to do.

Elliott is one of the author's own healthcare providers and a member of the neurology team that has been managing Ken's care throughout his migraine journey. His clinical contributions to this book reflect both his professional expertise and his firsthand understanding of the author's case — a perspective that bridges the gap between what the textbooks say and what actually happens in the exam room.

In his free time, Elliott enjoys spending time with his wife and kids, is a musician, and enjoys classic and modern literature. He did not, however, enjoy being asked to review this manuscript's snark level for clinical accuracy. He did it anyway, because that's the kind of amazing provider he is.

Made in the USA
Monee, IL
27 July 2026

58091744R00108